PREVENTABLE!

5 Powerful Practices to Avoid Disease and Build Unshakeable Health

Thomas Hemingway, M.D.

Editor: **Marjah Simon**

Author Writer's Academy (AWA)

Literary Agency, United States

www.AWA4Life.com

Cover Design, Illustrations, and Interior Layout by Author Writer's Academy

*For your <u>Free Powerful Daily Practices</u> PDF to accompany the mastery steps in this book, while available, visit <u>https://www.thomashemingway.com</u>

Dedication

To my grandfather, **Donald W. Hemingway**, who taught me from an early age that our health is largely up to us and under our control. He showed me there is so much we *can* do, and do so simply, as he taught me through his example of living a long, healthy, active life — well into his 90s, despite having insulin dependent diabetes the overwhelming majority of his life.

He always encouraged me to be curious and to ask lots of questions, to seek wisdom and knowledge no matter how much you already know, or think you know; and that the answers lie in the question, and in your humble ongoing pursuit of knowledge.

Thank you Grandpa; I love and miss you.

Table of Contents

Letter From the Author

You may have been told that the key to prevent or reverse disease or to lose weight is simply to go on a diet. Or perhaps you were told to eat less and exercise more.

Yet there is a better way.

No one should feel like they *have* to go on a diet. No one.

Diets often deprive and degrade. Most overwhelmingly fail. Ultimately, the data show the only consistent result of dieting is gaining weight in the long run.

So why is no one talking about this? Well, as many say, "Follow the money." Dieting is a multi-billion-dollar industry that almost all humans are familiar with. And indeed, most of us have likely tried at least one type of diet at some point in our lives.

If my aim was simply to make a bunch of money, I may have just written a diet book myself, or sold a diet plan or program. But for me, it is not about the money. It is about changing lives from the root of the matter. I want to make a *lifelong difference*, not simply add to the pile of quick fix and long-term failures of these superficial bandage solutions.

If you bought this book seeking yet another diet program, I am sorry to disappoint you.

> *This is NOT a diet book.*
> *It is instead a lifestyle approach to*
> *not only weight loss, but to*
> *achieving the health of your dreams.*

This book will share something bigger and much more effective than a diet. Instead of the hidden truth and undesirable near-guarantee of long-term weight gain — which almost all diets are prone to causing (but never tell you) — this approach has the potential to change your health and your life!

What I share will not only likely help you lose weight, but in fact enhance the quality of your *daily* life, while simultaneously adding years to it *overall*. I can't wait to share with you how this is possible.

It *is* doable, and the results can be phenomenal. All that is left now is to learn the principles here and then apply them!

Spoiler alert! No tasteless, regimented eating plans are prescribed here. Food is not only to nourish, but to ENJOY!

Eating can and should be something we look forward to, with a beaming smile from ear to ear! And by using the approach I share in this book, it can be precisely that. No diet or eating regimen should be dull, boring, tasteless, or without the simple joys and pleasures that come from eating delicious and nutritious real foods with those we love and care about!

So, *Bon Appetit!*
Thomas Hemingway, MD.

Introduction

It was six a.m. Monday morning. I just received word that a forty-nine-year-old man almost fainted in the hospital reception as he was checking in to the ER, where I work as a physician. He was immediately brought back to the treatment area. The patient, we will call him Henry, experienced sudden severe chest pain while getting ready for work that morning. For a moment, he later told me, he felt like he was going to die.

But then, the pain subsided, so he decided he would continue to get ready for work. Luckily for him, his wife had also been awakened by his alarm, and when she took one look at him knew that something was wrong. His blood seemed to have left his face, while he looked pale and sweaty, and altogether not quite right. She strongly encouraged him to get checked out at the local hospital. Yet he explained to me that he was reluctant to come to the hospital — it was Monday, a big day at the office, and the start of a busy work week for the company. But because he felt bad, being flushed, weak, and out of sorts, he acquiesced.

As a seasoned physician, his story was not unique to me. Heart attacks are extremely common, and heart disease is the number one cause of death worldwide for men and for women. In Henry's case, we were able to treat him with the state-of-the-art emergency care we are accustomed to providing, and, fortunately, he made a full recovery. Though this is not always the case. A significant number of first-time heart attack presentations end in sudden death or cardiac arrest. Of those who do survive, many lose significant heart function, which can dramatically limit their physical abilities in the future.

Heart disease is all too common in adult men and women between the ages of forty-five and sixty-five. It continues to be the number one cause of death in the United States, and in the developed world. In fact, heart attacks and cardiovascular problems cause at least one death every thirty-six seconds in the United States, and claim more than 650,000 lives per year. This amounts to one out of every four deaths in the U.S. Fortunately, it is almost entirely preventable. Yes, PREVENTABLE!

It's true, there *is* something that can be done about this — and it is much simpler than you might think.

One of the reasons I chose to write this book was to save lives. I do not intend to present ideas for a quick-fix diet, or a list of nutrition tips that may help you to lose a few pounds. Instead, this book contains powerful knowledge that can both prevent disease *and* save lives. Indeed, it may even save *yours*.

As a twenty-year veteran physician of emergency care, I have seen countless people die or suffer serious problems from heart disease. The sad fact, however, is that the majority of cases may have been delayed or prevented with simple nutrition and lifestyle modifications. It is these very changes that I will discuss in the forthcoming chapters of this book.

In Henry's case, though he was unaware of having prior health problems, he had known for a while that he needed to make changes to his food choices, and weight. He, like many of us, had set New Year's resolutions to lose weight and get healthy numerous times over the most recent decade of his life. The trouble was, he later told me, that although he would often have some initial success — losing a few pounds in the first couple of months of the year — he always struggled to keep it off. Ultimately, he would get frustrated, discouraged, and end up gaining more weight than his initial baseline.

After several attempts to try different dieting regimes, frequently resulting in "yo-yo" diet failures, he became even more discouraged, before finally giving up whatever diet and weight loss regimen he had chosen. As you will discover in this book, this scenario of following a diet plan to lose weight, having some early success, yet ultimately gaining more weight, is far too common.

Now, Henry's struggle with weight loss, however unsuccessful, is to be commended — he was trying to enact change. But because he was unaware of his high blood pressure, pre-diabetic status, high cholesterol, and insulin resistance prior to having a heart attack, the time spent following different fad diet plans would most likely have been better spent changing his lifestyle habits.

Weight loss is a challenge. Yet it is also only a *part* of the solution to better health. The goal of weight loss should be viewed as simply one element of a long-term strategy for optimal health, *not* a short-term solution.

> *I favor the goal of getting healthy to lose weight, over losing weight to get healthy.*

(Read that again.)

As you take the steps in this book to master the five powerful principles to regain your health, the weight loss you desire may happen concomitantly, and effortlessly.

Never forget — *There is hope!* There *is* something we can do to ensure long-term success — a fact that is based on physiology, and good science.

It is NOT your fault when you experience temporary weight loss, before long-term weight gain. It is instead one's physiology that factors into the speed of weight loss and later weight gain for the many who attempt to diet, and the subsequent choices we make that determine ultimate success. And you need not fret, as all of this will be revealed here, in this book!

I sincerely feel it is my responsibility, or *kuleana*, as we say in Hawaii, to share what I've learned from my decades-long experience as a physician and health advocate. We can each make a difference in our own life and the world by learning to live more healthily and vibrantly. And hopefully, in the end, we can also live largely free of these preventable health conditions that steal millions of lives each year around the world.

Did you know that at least seven out of ten of the leading causes of death in the U.S. and the developed world are preventable? Yes, you heard me correctly — PREVENTABLE. The most lethal, common, and costly health conditions that affect us as humans can be largely prevented by implementing the simple steps you will learn in this book.

Things do not have to be the way that they are right now, where we as a human race are perhaps the most unhealthy we have ever been. With obesity and diabetes rates rising rapidly across the globe; this *does not* have to be our destiny. We CAN change this. And I don't just wish this — I *know* something can be done. I have witnessed the results of these powerful preventative measures, and it starts right here, right now, with the information in this book.

Thankfully, the steps you can take to prevent these serious health problems are actually rather simple and uncomplicated. They are also both achievable and sustainable, and can prevent the top worldwide killers. I have seen this over and over with many who have changed the trajectory of their lives by applying the steps we will discuss in these pages. Just because you have certain genetics or a family history of a particular disease, you will soon learn that this does not have to be your future. Your future is instead largely in your own hands.

It is exhilarating to know that this power is within you, isn't it?

Yes, right here in this book, you will learn how you can improve your health, and maybe even drop a few pounds in the process, if that's what you desire. But most importantly, you will gain tools that may increase your life and health span, so that you can fully enjoy your time here on this planet. We only have *one life to live,* and it is my goal to help you make yours count!

My aim for the information I share is to help you get to a point where you are less likely to be limited by common debilitating and largely preventable health disorders and diseases. Health challenges such as; heart disease; cancer; stroke; Alzheimer's (and other dementias and neurodegenerative conditions); Type 2 diabetes; obesity, and most kidney diseases, can largely be prevented. And by following a few of the simple practices described right here in this book, you can be on your way to a more fruitful, vital, longer, and more enjoyable life.

If any of this interests you, read on!

Do you desire to spend extra years or even decades with your children, grandchildren, great-grandchildren, friends, pets, or other family members and other loved ones? Would you like to not only extend your physical life, but actually thrive, being truly present and vital to them for years to come? I know I would.

To help you do that, I want to share what I have discovered throughout my decades in medicine, health and wellness, and my own personal pursuit of optimal health.

First, we will identify the problem. Or specifically, the common threads to many preventable diseases. For once we have done this, we can then set our sights on treating them from the root cause. Now, this cannot simply be done by applying the proverbial superficial bandage, which too often most Western-trained physicians and practitioners attempt. Instead of attacking the root cause of the disease, symptoms are often treated with medication, as opposed to addressing the underlying cause. If we dig down to the root cause, we can potentially curtail and even prevent many of the contributing factors to premature deaths.

Did you know that it is estimated that the majority of people (over 50%) in the developed world are overweight, and as many as 88% are NOT metabolically healthy?[2] This staggering number, reported in a 2019 study, though hard to believe, is true. Furthermore, in recent years of the pandemic, I suspect these numbers have even gotten worse. In fact, my generation, and those that have followed, may have a shorter lifespan than even my own parents. Sadly, this is the first time in our lifetime and in more than the last 100 years of our history that the average lifespan in the developed world, especially in the U.S., is now decreasing, rather than increasing. The average lifespan was trending down even before the COVID-19 pandemic.[3]

So, what does being metabolically unhealthy mean? I will discuss this in detail throughout the book, though a few examples are those with diabetes; pre-diabetes; elevated body mass index; elevated lipids; high blood pressure; and insulin resistance. The latter of these, insulin resistance, is likely the most common metabolic health issue. Yet if you have any one of these afflictions, you may be considered metabolically unhealthy. Sadly, nearly 9/10 of us have one or more of these conditions, and many of us do not even know it. I know, I was one of them!

So, what are we doing about it?

In my humble opinion, not enough. We are missing the mark, and often starting late in the game (by ignoring, for example, mild elevations in blood sugar until they finally meet the diagnosis of full-blown diabetes).

My grandmother always told me, "An ounce of prevention is worth more than a pound of cure." This adage rings true now more than ever, with respect to our current health crisis: increasing rates of obesity, diabetes, heart disease, and many other chronic diseases. In fact, we have seen that the increasing rates of obesity have not only impacted the challenges we have faced during the pandemic, but in my experience also play into most chronic health conditions.

In this book, I will dive deep into explaining the physiology that impacts both weight loss and gain, and how to keep that gain at bay. I will also discuss how to avoid the common trend of repeated yo-yo dieting which many of us have experienced at some point in our lives.

Interestingly, dieting to some degree is more popular now than ever. It is a multibillion-dollar industry that has not proved to be a dependable solution. There are presently so many diets having little to no permanently positive results, and we, the people of the world, are getting fatter and fatter. The latest fad diets trending on social media are largely unsuccessful in the end. Indeed, the most common outcome of any dieting plan is a near-certain guarantee of future weight gain. This is good for the dieting business, but bad for us.

Given the lack of long-term success of most diets, the number of participants remains surprising. It is estimated that forty-five million people in the United States alone adopt diet plans each year.4 Optimistically, even though the lack of long-term success in dieting is a sad and common truth, I think it is commendable that people are positively trying to affect change in their lives. Unfortunately, however, this plan of action is clearly not a working solution to facilitate lasting health.

OK, a show of hands. Have you or someone you know ever been on a diet? If so, did it work long-term? Did you or that person lose the weight, and perhaps more importantly, keep it off? If your final answer is "no," you are not alone. This trend is so common that I would venture to call it the norm. So, if you have ever been on a diet, and couldn't keep the weight off long-term, I'd say you are normal.

Take a moment and let that sink in — YOU ARE NORMAL. Don't be hard on yourself, but instead have self-compassion, patience and give yourself grace. You will soon learn there is also a scientific reason why long-term weight loss through dieting is not easily attained. You are not weak, nor do you lack self-control — it is science. You are not to blame.

Take a deep breath now, and know that *you are enough,* and *not broken.*

The diets you may have tried are simply not set up to work long-term.

Many of us have at some point likely fallen into the group of "been there, done that" when it comes to dieting. According to the Center for Disease Control (CDC), as many as one in three adults diet at some point during any given year, and at least half of the adult population has tried to lose weight in the last twelve months.[5]

The reality that the majority of those who diet lose weight initially, but are unable to keep it off long-term, is daunting. I am not being pessimistic. Those who know me know that I am precisely the opposite. I am simply setting the stage for why dieting does not work long-term.

Another reason I decided to write this book is due, in part, to what I have witnessed over the last two decades as a physician. As a health and wellness educator, I have seen these dieting woes over and over again. As a doctor and an observer of my family, of my friends, and even their own, the reality that dieting does not seem to work as a long-term solution for weight loss has weighed heavily on me (no pun intended). This reality strikes very close to home, which I will explain shortly.

Dieting with no solid endgame has become so commonplace in my experience, and I feel obligated to share what I have learned in this area, in the hope that it will make your life better, healthier, happier, and even possibly extended. I come from a family where my mother, whom I love dearly, has felt pressured to be on a diet of some kind for the majority of her adult life. This equates to more than a half-century of dieting!

She has tried dozens of different programs, read dozens of books, and taken part in many classes and group sessions. She was often successful in her weight loss goals, but that success was repeatedly met with long-term struggles. For many reasons, my mother would alter her diet regime, return to previous habits, and thus struggle with dieting and nutritional goals for the better part of her life.

Many of the strategies she learned, as common as they are in the health and wellness space, are not based on good evidence, and have numerous flaws and weaknesses. The most damaging was to look at health goals through a short-term, diet goal lens. We should not be dieting, but instead making simple, yet significant, lasting lifestyle changes.

Now, I do not pretend to have every answer to every question about dieting or weight loss, or optimal health. But I *have* learned a variety of fundamental principles that are well-founded in science, *and* have produced undeniable results in both my own life and those of countless others. With this, I cannot express how privileged I feel touching the lives of many during my own journey in health and wellness.

I am not the typical Western-trained medical doctor who, though largely well-meaning, tends to reach for the prescription pad. Many doctors often treat medical issues according to the symptoms and ailments presented by their patients after spending a cursory few minutes with them in the exam room, or perhaps more recently via a teleconference call.

This brief "bandage," symptom-based and reductionist approach ("the pill for every ill approach") typically fails to achieve real lasting health changes, because it frequently does not address the root cause of the medical issue. I believe what is at the end of our forks holds more power to heal than most prescription medications. I believe *food is medicine* (more on this later in the book).

Generally, it is not that the medical professional lacks skill in approaching ailments from a root cause point of view, but that they are not uniformly taught to use this approach.

Instead, they are typically trained to diagnose and treat based on symptoms.

Handing out pharmaceutical prescriptions is often a knee-jerk treatment tool response. So, the fault does not rest squarely on the shoulders of doctors who perform in this manner. They simply perform the duties of their profession in the way that they were trained.

How do I know? I've been there. This traditional "band-aid" approach to medical treatment often focuses on tending to a symptom or problem superficially. As physicians, we often swiftly treat without necessarily digging for the root cause(s). Yet if these are appropriately discovered and addressed, it may preclude any need for medication altogether.

My experience has led me to believe that less is often more if we implement a few simple actions correctly and repeatedly over time. Treatment in the form of new medication often complicates and clouds one's picture of health. The pharmaceutical approach may even make matters worse, as most medications have numerous and potentially serious side effects. Moreover, when new medications are combined with others that an individual may already be taking (termed "poly-pharmacy"), the potential for adverse reactions increases significantly.

It is not uncommon for a physician to prescribe additional medications to treat the side effects of the other medications a patient is taking (I know, I have seen this often and have done this myself in my early practice.) Yet this is merely "adding fuel to the fire." Considering our oath as physicians to *first, do no harm*, I believe compliance with this promise encompasses the healing process we need to practice in treating our patients in a manner that ensures a positive path to good health.

To expand on my point, have you ever seen a commercial about the latest medication for a certain digestive disorder or skin condition? The suggestion often follows that, if you take this medication, you will be cured. After showing numerous images of happily treated patients (actors), the commercial will then list dozens and dozens of potentially severe side effects (including things like heart attack, stroke, severe infection, immune compromise, and even death). The truth is, many of these disorders and conditions are preventable and treatable *without* medications, by merely taking steps toward attaining and maintaining a healthy lifestyle. In my humble opinion, risking liver failure, immune system compromise, sepsis and potentially death to treat your skin condition, does not seem like a wise trade-off.

As a physician, I have personally seen dozens of patients suffer from severe side effects from medications, of all classes. Some are life-threatening, and others even fatal. It is truly heartbreaking, so I do not reflect upon this lightly or without deep thought and concern. I know many patients really need these medications. Though I also believe the physician who prescribed them is likely doing what he or she feels is best, with no malice or intent to cause harm.

That being said, the reality is that each prescribed medication has the potential to cause harm — just read the label or package insert. Should this not at least give us pause in determining their overall use and long-term effect on our health? Considering this, should we not seek safer, non-pharmacologic treatment options, when available?

Many people do not know that side effects and errors relating to medication and medical treatments are a leading cause of death in the developed world, AND are preventable! This is not something most physicians will ever discuss or acknowledge with their patients — the notion that medical treatment may cause harm. In fact, recent data from PubMed suggests that medical errors may be the 3rd leading cause of death in the United States, accounting for 251,000 unnecessary deaths annually in the U.S. alone.[6]

Now, this is not a book on medical treatment or prescription management for any particular disease, symptom, or health disorder, nor is it a diagnosis and treatment approach to any particular condition. In fact, this book is not medical advice of any kind, and should not replace any ongoing relationship with your personal healthcare provider. It is, instead, written for educational and entertainment purposes only (with a heavier focus on the former, if you catch my drift).

I will try, for the most part, to avoid writing too much about any specific medications, as I recommend you have these discussions with your own personal physician or healthcare provider. Instead, I want to give you a broad understanding of many important health and wellness principles. If followed, these may lead you to a healthier, happier, and more energetic YOU. Crucially, this will allow you to have the ability to live your life less restrained by many of the very common and often preventable health ailments we increasingly face as a society each day.

I will be the first to admit that I am not perfect with all of my health choices. Although, by nature, my personality is such that I have struggled with the so-called curse of perfectionism for most of my life. This is to say I have been really hard on myself with many things, including my health choices, over the years. I eventually realized that this behavior had often been both unproductive and counterproductive. Like you, in seeking better health practices, I fell victim to the constant rollercoaster of fad dieting and other *en vogue* health practices.

Rather than be a perfectionist with respect to healthy eating, I have come to endorse what I like to loosely call the "80:20" rule. This is to say that 80% of the time I strive to make great healthy eating and nutrition decisions, and 20% of the time may indulge in some perhaps not-so-perfect foods or behaviors. Sometimes, I may even shoot for a 90:10 rule, but my personal minimum goal is 80:20. Yet this is certainly not where I started.

An example to demonstrate this would be dessert. Usually I opt out of having desserts (after meals), but if I am celebrating my kids' birthdays (like I do at least six times a year!), I may eat a small slice of cake. But I make the choice to not go for seconds. I endorse this, because in my experience if we are too rigid with our dietary choices, it may prove difficult to maintain goals long-term (like most diets). It may also easily detract from our enjoyment of both food and life.

The last thing I want for myself, or you, is to feel like we are living a deprived or restricted life, without the pleasures of enjoying tasty, delectable foods, and good company. Ask anyone who knows me, and they will tell you that I love to eat, often described as a "good eater." I simply love good food, and most importantly, have found that one can eat tasty foods AND be healthy!

Beyond this simple, 80:20 rule, I like to add another powerful rule of 80. This is something I have learned from studying the longest lived people in the world, in this specific example, the people of Okinawa, Japan. Here they have the saying, "Hara hachi bu," which means to eat until you are 80% full. In other words, don't eat until you are stuffed, satiated and feel full as I used to after Thanksgiving or Christmas dinner, or after eating at my favorite restaurant. Instead, eat until you are just 80% full or just starting to feel satisfied.

What has helped me here is to eat a bit more slowly, savoring the individual bites of tasty food, chewing more, and then stopping when I start to feel satisfied, rather than necessarily finishing my plate, as at a restaurant, for example. This way I not only feel better after my meal as I don't feel "stuffed to the gills" and desiring a nap, but still feel up for my favorite post-meal activity, taking a walk, which further aids my digestion and metabolic health.

In this fashion I have eaten plenty of tasty foods — at home, eating out, or at a holiday party — while staying healthy. Eating delicious foods and being healthy are not mutually exclusive, thank goodness! In fact, one of my favorite vacations of all time, which was almost twenty years ago, was a trip I took with my wife to Italy, where we enjoyed some of the best food I have ever eaten in my entire life! Yes, we also saw some amazing places with major historical significance, but the part I enjoyed most was the simple, real, wholesome, and extremely tasty home-cooked food we enjoyed there on a daily basis.

Just thinking about this makes my mouth water, testament to how much I enjoyed the Mediterranean cuisine. I will touch on this enjoyment more when I discuss the Mediterranean and other real food ways of eating, later in the book. But for now, just remember that the notion of living a healthy and enjoyable life while eating wonderful food is possible!

How else do you think those centenarians from Italy have been able to live beyond one hundred years, and still maintain their senses and enjoy their lives tremendously? It is the home-cooked, real food they regularly consume, and the connection they have with their family and community. The fact that many Italians don't practice some of the harmful behaviors we have in the West (such as our sedentary lifestyles and diets rich in processed foods) is a further example.

You will see throughout this book that my approach is generally *prevention over prescription*. This is not my approach alone, but is one that is shared by many holistic, integrative, and functional medicine providers, and has its roots in the Hippocratic Oath I took in the 1990s. The most important part of the oath — "Do no harm."

Interestingly enough, a lesser known passage of the Hippocratic Oath, which directly precedes the promise to do no harm, states, "I will use those dietary regimens which will benefit my patients according to my greatest ability and judgment."[7] This is in perfect alignment with my intent for this book, because:

Food truly is medicine.
So, before you dig in, take a deep breath,
celebrate yourself for having the desire
to take charge of your health and your life,
and set aside any insecurities
or negative self-talk
about how much you
may have struggled until now.
This is a journey and a lifestyle change,
not a final destination
or goal post-event,
which may change
the trajectory of your life forever.
Are you ready?

CHAPTER 1

Dieting in the Face of the Worst Obesity Epidemic in Human History

> *"If you don't do what's best for your body,*
> *you're the one who comes up on the short end."*
> **—Julius Erving "Dr. J"**

Many of you have likely experienced that dieting, for the most part, does not yield the positive results you seek for lasting success. Why? Well, there are many reasons. To start with, for better or worse, there is a growing understanding that dieting alone does not result in sustainable weight loss, because we focus too much on short-term results, rather than long-term health.

But don't worry! If you have previously sailed on this boat, and the diet you chose did not work out as planned, you are normal!

A very interesting article in the prestigious *British Medical Journal*, published in April of 2020, confirms this observation: that most diets do not result in long-term weight loss. In fact, it contains a robust collection of data from nearly 22,000 patients, concluding, "Overall, weight loss diminished at twelve months among all macronutrient patterns and popular named diets. Moderate certainty evidence shows that most macronutrient diets over six months result in modest weight loss and improvements in cardiovascular risk factors, particularly blood pressure. However, at twelve months the effects on weight reduction and improvements in cardiovascular risk factors largely disappear."[8]

Effects on weight reduction and positive heart benefits disappear at twelve months? Yes, you heard that right! For the overwhelming majority of us, this is what happens, and you may have experienced this with one of the many diets out there. Do you now see why I believe and suggest that dieting does not work in the long-term? If this has ever been you, take a breath and have compassion for yourself. This is the norm. Your experiences are normal. *There is nothing wrong with you.*

This was a large, systematic review and meta-analysis (a study where the researchers combined data from multiple scientific studies). In this case, they analyzed 121 dieting trials that enrolled nearly 22,000 overweight or obese adults who followed one of fourteen popular diets: Atkins, Weight Watchers, Jenny Craig, DASH, Mediterranean diet, and others, for an average of six months.

The diets were grouped into one of three categories: low-carbohydrate, low-fat, and moderate-macronutrient (diets in this category were similar to those in the low-fat group, but with slightly more fat and slightly fewer carbohydrates). Loss of both excess weight and cardiovascular measures (including cholesterol and blood pressure) while following one of these diets was compared with other diets or usual diets (one in which the person continued to eat as they normally would).

While weight, blood pressure, and cholesterol measures generally improved at the six-month mark (after the participants observed the respective diets consistently for six months), results at the twelve month mark were disappointing, to say the least. While the low-carb and low-fat diets both resulted in weight loss of about ten pounds at the six-month mark, most of the lost weight, unfortunately, was regained within one year.

Similar short-term gains showed a modest improvement in blood pressure and cholesterol at six months, but these also returned to their beginning levels after one year. One exception was noted, however. Reduced low-density lipoproteins (LDL) cholesterol levels while on the Mediterranean diet persisted for one year. Finally, the study concluded there were no major differences in other health benefits between the various diet programs.

Disappointing, is it not? Particularly given that this was a large data set, with over 22,000 participants in many popular diet programs. Yet most of the participants could not keep the weight off that they lost at the one-year mark.

Another study, this time from *Medical Clinics of North America* in 2018, followed twenty-nine long-term weight loss studies, and showed that more than half of the lost weight was regained within two to five years. And by five years, more than 80% of lost weight was regained.[9] These data show a lot!

What should not surprise you is the need that many dieting programs have for repeat customers. If you fail once, you choose another. Then another, and another. According to the *Research and Markets* study reported in February 2019, the U.S. weight loss market alone is worth a record $72 billion dollars![10]

Remember those plans you made for better health and a smaller waist size at the top of the year? Dieting plans thrive on New Year's resolutions. Nearly half (48%) of those who made New Year resolutions in 2019 wanted to lose weight, according to a survey by YouGov.[11] My humble conclusion: for those who are interested in losing weight, and keeping it off, there is a more effective plan than simply following a popularized diet.

Almost no one who sets out with a goal plans to fail. Not you, not me. I don't believe dieting to be any different. Each and every year nearly half of goal-setters want to lose weight. No judgment here, but most of us fail at this in the long-term. Yet I am confident we can change this! In order to do so, however, we need to do something *different*. As Einstein is often quoted as saying, "Insanity is doing the same thing over and over again and expecting a different result." This very notion has been proven in research on dieting and weight loss time and again. It is uncommon that long-term weight loss from dieting can be maintained.[12]

As you may have guessed, I am not a fan of dieting. I am specifically not in favor of one or more of the numerous fad diets out there that seem to reinvent themselves year after year. By the numbers, too many of us have attempted, on far too frequent an occasion, any number of dieting plans, and long-term success has often eluded us.

Thus, my intent with this book is to discuss how lasting weight loss and improved health can happen, without necessarily following any of the popular diets out there. My belief is that most of us actually want results that will last, and not merely a quick fix to a persistent problem. We want a lasting and impactful plan that changes our lives for the better. Better health, for a longer and more fulfilled life. Does this sound like you?

Dieting, you will quickly see, has many fallacies, inconsistencies, and conundrums. I will explain a selection of the more common ones, and how to avoid getting stuck in these proverbial tar pits, in the chapters to come. With this, I will use health principles, minus the dogma, and show how we can apply these concepts to achieve weight loss (if desired) and improved overall health. Knowing these principles will then help you avoid some of the most common illnesses or diseases responsible for much of the rising morbidity and mortality rates to date. Ultimately, our endgame should be to live better, and hopefully longer.

Let's take a deeper dive now, using data from the CDC, with respect to the scope of the problem that fuels our common desire to diet or simply lose weight. Yes, I am going to talk about being overweight and obese. Yet I do so objectively, and without any judgment, in order to simply put into context the severity and breadth of this issue. The numbers are quite staggering, and sadly predicted to worsen in the coming years — *unless* we do something about it. If we don't change our trajectory, none of this changes.

Fortunately, however, we *can* change this. And it can be quite simple.

Recent data from the CDC shows how common obesity is today, having increased in the recent decade. It is reported that the age-adjusted prevalence of obesity among U.S. adults was 42.4% in 2017–2018.[13] The prevalence was 40.0% among younger adults aged 20–39, 44.8% among middle-aged adults aged 40-59, and 42.8% among older adults aged 60 and over. There were no significant differences in prevalence by age group (i.e., all adults in this group from age 20 to over 60 had similar levels of obesity). Almost one-half of them! A heavy increase from just 15 years prior, when in 2002, 25.6% of U.S. adults were classified as obese by the CDC.

Now you may ask yourself, what exactly does obesity mean, and how does it compare to being overweight? (Hint — obesity is worse than simply being overweight.) A much higher percentage of us will classify as being overweight: nearly 71% in the U.S., as of 2016.[14] Yet how do we define overweight and obese? Well, this is defined rather simply by the CDC, in terms related to the body mass index (BMI). Let me explain, with an example from their website.

BMI is a person's weight in kilograms divided by the square of their height in meters.[15] In other words, it is a numerical value obtained by knowing your weight and height — it is that simple. A high BMI can be an indicator of high body fat, if you will. This is not necessarily the best measurement of body fat or obesity, though it is frequently used worldwide, and thus can be used for comparison purposes as it is the most common method used in the reported literature.

To calculate BMI, see the Adult BMI Calculator, or determine your BMI by finding your height and weight in a BMI chart.

- If your BMI is less than 18.5, it falls within the underweight range.
- If your BMI is 18.5 to <25, it falls within the normal range.
- If your BMI is 25.0 to <30, it falls within the overweight range.
- If your BMI is 30.0 or higher, it falls within the obese range.[16]

Let us look at an example:

Here is John. He wants to know his BMI, and knows he is five foot eight inches (1.73 meters) tall and weighs 190 pounds (86.2 kilograms). To calculate his BMI, we would divide 86.2

by (1.73 x 1.73). A simple calculation would yield a result of 28.9 for his BMI, which would classify him as overweight.

This helps us to understand the magnitude of the problem, because obesity is defined as being significantly overweight to the tune of a BMI greater than 30. In our example, John is approaching this with his BMI at nearly 29 (while just being overweight is having a BMI over 25).

Simply stated, despite some of our contributions to a 72 billion dollar diet industry, Americans continue to get fatter and fatter. From 1999–2000 through 2017–2018, the age-adjusted prevalence of obesity increased from 30.5% to 42.4%, and the prevalence of severe obesity increased from 4.7% to 9.2%.[13]

Becoming overweight or obese has now reached epidemic proportions (71% and 42.4% in 2018, respectively). This begs the question, "What are we going to do about it?"

Well, we CAN change our trajectory.

Yet first, we must understand where and how this phenomenon began, before making healthy plans to change it. Ours, our family's, and our world's future health depend on it.

This issue is not merely important because it's common. That is just the tip of the iceberg. It is also important because the significant health ramifications have quite literally become a matter of life and death. The majority of the top ten most common causes of death,17 as mentioned in the introduction, are exacerbated by and tend to coexist alongside obesity — heart disease, cancer, diabetes, stroke, lower respiratory illness, COVID-19, and kidney disease. These conditions tend to be more common in overweight and obese patients.

Not only will one be more likely to have significant health problems if obese, but beyond that, studies show obesity by itself can shorten one's lifespan. I saw this first-hand during my time as a medical student on the surgery rotation in the 1990s. I worked with a bariatric surgeon for several months, and we routinely treated patients of more than 200kg (440lbs). On several occasions, I examined patients in their own homes or a rented van, as they were unable to sit or stand on their own, or ride in a typical vehicle.

Their quality of life was severely affected, and it was not uncommon to hear of their early exit from this life in their 30s and 40s. This was heartbreaking, and it prompted me to pursue additional studies into natural and root cause approaches, in order to help with their condition. Although surgery was often partially effective in the short-term, it seemed rare in bringing them the weight loss they desired in the long run.

According to the prestigious *Journal of the American Medical Association* (JAMA), as reported in November of 2018, data from the well-known Framingham study tracked the weight and survival of more than 6,000 Americans for 24 years, and found that obesity can lead to early death.[18] Obesity (BMI between 30-34) was tied to a 27% increase in the odds of dying within the study period, and the risk of dying young was even higher for the very obese (those with a BMI of 35 to 39). People in this weight category had nearly double the odds of dying during the study period, compared to people with a normal weight.

This is reason alone to give pause, wouldn't you agree? Statistically, many of us (up to 42.4% of adults) will likely live shorter lives due in part to obesity and related problems. I don't know about you, but for me, more than anything, I want to see my kids grow up. I want to see my children's children grow up. Furthermore, I would humbly submit that not only is it the length of life that should interest us (any biohackers out there?), but also the quality of life.

It seems natural to propose that quality of life will also be affected by obesity. And this has indeed been demonstrated by a 2015 Brazilian study. It showed obesity contributed to a measurable decrease in quality of life for the obese individual.[19]

Now that we have established that obesity is truly an epidemic, affecting over 42% of the U.S. population and millions worldwide, let's put this in perspective. Being overweight and obese has now surpassed both worldwide hunger and starvation in its respective prevalence throughout the world. At the same time, it now surpasses other health challenges both in sheer numbers and its negative health consequences, making it an extremely costly epidemic.

According to a report from the prestigious medical journal *The Lancet*, obesity is now the leading cause of disabilities globally.[20] According to this report, every country, with the exception of sub-Saharan Africa, is facing an alarming increase in obesity rates — 82% globally in the past two decades. Even Middle Eastern countries have high obesity rates, seeing an astounding 100% increase since 1990. Here in the U.S., we have one of the highest obesity rates in the entire world.

Is it hard to imagine that our ancestors did not experience this problem? Over the last several decades, obesity has become a prevalent thorn in our health system, which is only projected to get worse within the decade. Unless, of course, we change this. Yet I propose we can, and we must.

Part of this will involve taking a step back to the way we used to eat, before unhealthy, excessive, non-nutritive, highly processed, calorically dense, and nutritionally poor food became a part of the health crisis that persists today. No, obesity is not an epidemic from the past. It is a new phenomenon; the curse of prosperity and convenience.

Yes, being overweight, and to a greater extent being obese, pose significant health problems, comorbidities, and higher mortality rates. The quality of your life on a day-to-day basis is dramatically affected, as well as its ultimate length. So, you may ask, how did we get here, and what can be done about it?

This is where I'd like to place our attention and focus within this book. A lot can be done about this circumstance. We are not victims. This health crisis does not ravage indiscriminately, and we *can* do something about it.

Certain choices we have made as a society have brought us here. Yet different choices will see us through to a healthier future. And sure, we can do something about this, but this needs to become a MUST.

By definition, "preventable" inherently means that we can affect the outcome. And indeed, we can turn this worldwide epidemic around — this is what is so exciting! You cannot begin to imagine how much this motivates me to share!

Indeed, this is how my book differs from the abundance of common dieting books out there. This is not about a fad diet, gimmick, or cutesy rehashed way to try to lose weight. This book may actually teach you lifelong strategies on how to achieve your ideal health and weight, achievements which will not be fleeting and temporary, but instead might last a lifetime! And, believe it or not, it will not require any lengthy lists or calorie counting. *Say what?*

Read on, and you will soon learn how we got here (how obesity came to be so prevalent), and why dieting typically fails to promote long-term weight loss.

After this, you will learn a variety of simple, easy to implement foundational principles for HOW we get healthy, lose weight naturally, and do so without dieting at all!

So, let's go!

CHAPTER 2

Dieting Does Not Work...

> *"I always believed if you take care of your body*
> *it will take care of you."*
> **–Ted Lindsay**

Let us begin with one powerful reason for why diets do not work. They are naturally a restriction, and fight against every instinct we have as human beings. As humans, we often rebel against restrictions. For example, how many of us obey the speed limit *100% of the time*, or *always* remained inside during recent quarantines? Unfortunately, I didn't. Human nature demands that we take a walk, visit friends and relatives, or go connect with people. Being deprived of our human nature and right to connect restricted our lives in ways we were not prepared, for example.

Diets are also restrictive. Eliminating processed and fried foods, dairy, sugar, gluten, and many convenience or comfort foods from the normal dietary "menu" can be a restriction. Most people are not thrilled about the restrictive nature of diets, no matter the promise of a smaller waistline. Be honest. You don't *enjoy* depriving yourself of things that bring you happiness, right? The restrictive nature of diets is a major reason people tend to quit their regimes shortly after starting.

Food is fundamental to our enjoyment of life, in mind, spirit, and body. So let's enjoy it!

Eating good food can be a true joy, and taking the pleasure out of it through unnecessary or overly restrictive dieting will make it next to impossible to continue. No one likes feeling restricted — certainly not me, and I am sure you feel the same. I certainly don't recommend depriving yourself of the *joy* of eating. Why would you want to? And in the following chapters, you will learn that you don't have to!

For now, however, I want to continue to explore additional ways dieting is not a sustainable method for losing weight or reaching your optimal health goals. We will begin by looking at whether dieting is a solution for long-term health. Is it the answer to achieving our best body and health status? Can dieting actually help us achieve and maintain our health goals?

Let's jump in, and discuss it all!

For Lifelong Health

Most of us intuitively know that dieting does not reliably and uniformly produce lasting lifestyle changes. Depending on the diet, it may be quite difficult to maintain certain required actions long-term. Therefore, most dieters fall short of continuing their program for the duration. The average person may find sustaining the menu and rules on a day-to-day basis difficult, which then becomes a key factor in any unsuccessful long-term outcome.

For the most part, this is precisely why I do not recommend dieting, nor do I recommend calorie counting — a common denominator among most diets. From personal and shared experience, I can honestly say the mechanics of calorie counting alone do not lend significant benefit towards enabling optimal health and long-term weight loss.

Don't just take my word for it — refer to the data. One of the largest systematic reviews of numerous dieting studies (a meta-analysis) conducted by researchers at UCLA found that only a small percentage of the individuals who employed a dieting strategy (commonly using a conventional calorie-restricted diet) were able to actually lose weight and keep it off over time.[21]

Furthermore, the UCLA researchers have indicated that the act of dieting by itself is actually one of the best predictors of future weight gain, not weight loss.[21] Janet Tomiyama, one of the UCLA study's authors, reviewed the data, which included

31 separate dieting studies, and concluded that dieting is actually a very consistent predictor of future weight gain.

Yet another study reviewed by these UCLA researchers was of obese patients who were followed for varying lengths of time throughout their dieting regime.[21] Among those who were followed for less than two years, 23% gained back more weight than they had lost. Of the group who were followed for at least two years, 83% regained more weight than they had lost. One study even found that 50% of those dieters gained more than eleven pounds over their starting weight five years after the diet. Yikes!

Overall, not only does the data show that dieting does not result in sustainable weight loss, but that it also most often predicts future weight *gain*, in excess of that lost while dieting.

To summarize, diets do not generally result in lasting weight loss. In fact, they seem to have the opposite effect long-term, frequently leading to future weight gain. More than half of the U.S. population have tried dieting to lose weight, but with these attempts come an overwhelming majority who have not succeeded in sustaining long-term weight loss — still with me?

Based on these studies, you *may* be tempted to throw in the towel on your dieting goals altogether, but please don't! There's another way of looking at this. It seems to matter less which plan you pick (whether low-carb, low-fat, Keto, Paleo, vegan, vegetarian, carnivore, or something in between) than if you *stick with* those action plans and continue the dietary behaviors long-term.

My favorite explanation for the pitfalls of dieting is that the word "DIET" has the word "DIE" in it. And no one wants to "die," right?! So why would we want to diet? Even so, many of us think we ought to diet, in order to lose "x" amount of weight, which could be for any number of personal reasons, such as health conditions, to feel better, fit into that perfect dress or jeans, impress others, and so on.

When people ask me what exercise is best for them,
I simply respond,
"The one that you will do, and do consistently,
over the long haul."
Similarly, with dieting and overall healthy eating,
the health plan that you will actually put in place
and sustain long-term will likely be the one I recommend.

Rather than follow a highly restrictive diet, I personally follow a "whole food or real food" diet, that is probably best described as a cross between the Keto, Paleo, and Mediterranean diets — chock-full of nutritious, and believe me, delicious food. I, in no way, deprive myself. Nor can I ever prescribe, or promote, any specific dietary plan that does not have healthy, tasty, and real food. What you will learn right here in this book is that tasty and healthy are *not* mutually exclusive!

Would you continue with a juicing diet that consisted of repeatedly juicing kale if you do not like the taste? Not likely. If quinoa is your least favorite food, would you follow a plan that insisted you eat it every day? Of course not. If you can't stand the menu in the short-term, you likely won't continue it in the long run.

Ultimate benefits lie in the continuity of diet and healthy eating choices for years — this is where the magic happens. It is your choices that lead to a true lifestyle change, as you aim for your new routine of a healthier lifestyle to become effortless and a part of your daily living. You can *enjoy* and *love* the food you eat, and it can *love* you back.

This is where the process gets exciting — when we pick the foods and behaviors that are both healthy and enjoyable. By doing this, we actually create a space for ourselves through which to continue these behaviors long-term. When our health plan is built with foods that are both healthy and enjoyable to us, coupled with behaviors we also design from healthy options, positive benefits follow. We are much more likely to continue with healthy behavior and a healthy eating plan long-term if we pick the foods and the activities ourselves; not by following diet rules from a program.

Here, I would like to give you an example:

This is the case of Jim, a middle-aged man who begins a particularly regimented diet consisting of eating kale twice a day, and other foods he does not find particularly appealing. In the process, he discovers how much he can't stand the taste of kale. Nevertheless, he initially proceeds with the regimen, and manages to stick with the program for 4 weeks, losing 14 pounds. He cannot, in a million years, fathom the idea of eating kale as part of his long-term diet.

After a month, he quits the program, and not long after returns to his previous habits of eating pre-packaged, processed, and fast food, and swiftly regains the weight — plus an additional 5 pounds! Indulgence becomes his norm once again, and the discipline he practiced those 4 weeks flies out the window. Now, this is not an extreme case, but common. It is often the theme tying together the many reasons why diets fail in the long run.

Case studies performed by nutritional experts; patient cases documented by health practitioners; and witnessing family and friends struggle with choices that fail to have long-term positive results have all added to my understanding of the issue. These all represent what we can learn about the power of making healthy choices that are comfortable for our individual selves. When you make a comfortable choice for yourself, and the right choice for your body from the very beginning of your lifestyle change, you will have a higher success rate of reaching your goals and attaining long-term health.

In addition to the emphasis on quality whole foods, there are a variety of other factors that can have a big impact on weight and long-term health. For example, everyday physical activity, like regular cardiovascular exercise and strength training, adequate quality sleep, stress optimization, and focusing on gut health, are all very important in helping maintain a healthy weight and optimal health.

Indeed, our behavior when seeking optimal health must go beyond simply what we put into our mouths. Although what we eat is both paramount and foundational; optimal health, wellness, and achieving our ideal weight all have multiple contributors. And as you read on, you will come to learn a lot about these other avenues as well which together makeup the five powerful practices to focus on in order to avoid disease and achieve optimal health.

If taken together, the action plans throughout will provide you with the best chance of achieving long-term health, wellness, and weight loss. For now, though, let us first explore some other factors of why traditional dieting can be problematic.

Because it is Too Heavy Psychologically

The restrictive nature of diets can often cause a negative psychological impact for those who attempt them and fall short of their goals. This very restriction contributes to our desire to rebel. To take control of this restriction, or to feel some sense of normalcy under abnormal circumstances, we create a space that allows us to enjoy ourselves. This comes in the form of a "cheat day," which is often molded into the structure of many diets.

This is normal, and certainly understandable! I do have one suggestion, however: do not allow your "cheat days" to lead you back to where you started. It is a slippery downhill spiral if you are not careful how you manage these days. This can then lead to some of the other negative consequences of dieting, potentially harming your psychological health and well-being due to feelings of guilt, shame, embarrassment, and unworthiness.

Let's imagine a case where someone begins a diet with optimism and enthusiasm, a real "I'm going to do it this time" attitude. "I'm ready!" to lose weight, and fit into those clothes I've been wanting to get back into for so long. With this optimism and motivation, the person loses a few pounds in the first two weeks. This initial success is enough to keep him or her motivated to press on, in hopes their weight loss will continue. But this does not happen.

Yet why? Well, what followed was the realization that after speedy weight loss at the beginning of a diet, such loss tends to plateau. When we stop losing weight at the speed we desire, our optimism wanes, we get frustrated with the process, and slowly we begin justifying that extra handful of potato chips or other comfort food. Beyond this, if we practice a certain degree of caloric restriction, our body adjusts to this and may begin to hold onto the calories more strongly, making it far harder to lose additional weight.

This can lead to even more frustration, making us feel guilty about not succeeding with our diet the way we desired. We may begin to feel sad, not good enough, mad, or even depressed. Do we throw in the towel, though? No, not yet. We do not quit altogether. But how do we deal with those feelings of guilt, sadness, and frustration?

We may turn these frustrations into a "cheat" day. That alluring "cheat" meal. The dopamine release in the brain these provide, giving us that rush of pleasure associated with satisfying a craving or desire, quells the feelings of sadness, frustration, and depression. But is a "cheat day" the answer? Is it the best way to keep us motivated to continue engaging with our set dietary menu, and help us reach our weight loss goal?

Cheat days compound the bigger issue of unhealthy lifestyles. The very lifestyles that lead to gaining weight in the first place. Also, think about it — one cheat day can lead to another, only this time a bigger cheat. Bigger cheats lead to binges. And binges eventually lead you *back* to weight gain. One "cheat" simply brings about another. And so on. Are you getting the picture now? This common cycle of weight loss, followed by weight gain, on repeat, is often coined the vicious cycle of yo-yo dieting.

Now, this is not to shame, guilt, cause feelings of unworthiness, or anything else to those of you out there. This is science! And more specifically, neurobiology. This yo-yo effect can be explained by the release of dopamine in the pleasure centers of the brain in response to craving and eating foods we find enjoyable. This euphoria occurs in a similar area and by a similar mechanism in the brain that euphoric drugs such as cocaine and amphetamines stimulate.

Once this temporary pleasure dissipates, what follows is heightened feelings of frustration, shame, and even despair. Remember that extra handful of potato chips? To assuage the guilt from eating off the dietary menu, your pleasure center shouts, "Why not have more?! Go on, it'll make you feel better!" To which a repetitive cycle of unhealthy eating ensues. Yo-yo dieting lands us right back at the deprivation stage of dieting, followed by a self-imposed pleasure day, which will likely lead us back to the same unhealthy practices that produced our initial weight gain.

What you need to understand is that this is truly not an issue of willpower or lack of self-control, but physiology. This cycle is simply a normal reaction to a process forced upon you by the pre-packaged and processed food industry to create tasty, difficult-to-resist, addictive products that boost sales. Methodically adhered to by nearly all of the big food companies for at least the last several decades (likely much longer), this process keeps us hooked on tasty, seemingly irresistible, but ultimately unhealthy products.22

It may be a surprise to you that certain foods (especially those that are highly processed, sweet, or salty [junk food]) have been purposefully designed in a laboratory by specially trained food scientists, to trigger the dopamine rush in the brain that leaves us craving and desiring more. But this is common knowledge in the world of health and wellness. Millions and millions of dollars are spent in food science labs, creating ways to get us hooked on these highly processed foods, and boosting sales while contributing to the biggest obesity epidemic in our world's history.22

There is no place for shame here, as it is not only demeaning and hurtful but very counterproductive. What I teach is that desiring junk food is a normal reaction when forcing other dietary restrictions upon our bodies. Therefore, do not feel ashamed for giving in to that *urge to splurge*. You are normal for desiring what you have committed to not consume. Our cravings are supplemented by the specific engineering of those foods, which means it may be hard to resist them! This is not in any way a sign of a loss of self-control or a lack of willpower — it's science! So stop shaming yourself! Now!

> *You are enough,*
> and *you are not broken.*

Over time, this cycle of starting and stopping and starting again, diet after diet, can be extremely detrimental to our mental, physical, and psychological health. Our feeling of self-worth is dented each time we fail at a new diet. I humbly submit that this may indeed be another reason why diets don't work. Dieting is certainly not how I recommend going about a lifestyle change. The psychological pressure of succeeding at a regimen that is more short-term results-driven, as opposed to a long-term, healthful outlook, presents an unnecessary negative toll on one's mental health. The guilt or shame you may feel by not successfully reaching your weight goal often leads to more weight gain. Indeed, a downhill spiral is an unnatural, yet predictable, dividend of dieting.

I think this psychological component often goes undiscussed and underemphasized in many dieting techniques, and, in my experience, often in the medical and wellness spaces. Moreover, because I have witnessed how significantly it impacts many people's lives, I have decided to mention here how important psychological wellness is to a lifestyle change. Its role in dieting plays a major part in positive and negative outcomes. It is also an important feature of overall health and wellness. It is empowering to understand its nuances, while this wellness can easily be applied to successful changes in lifestyle.

I want you to know, with every fiber of your being, that YOU ARE CAPABLE, GOOD ENOUGH, and WORTHY to make your lifestyle change work. You CAN make long-standing changes to your health, weight, and life. And, you CAN choose to do this right now! It does NOT have to be difficult. We will go into certain practices later in the book that will demonstrate this. For they are not only healthful, beneficial, and life-changing, but simple, making success possible for each and every one of us! Remember, *you are enough and you are not broken.* Your metabolism, on the other hand, may be broken and not currently operating at full efficiency. However, as you will find later in the book, this can quite easily and quickly be fixed with simple and sustainable practices detailed herein.

For the most part, these steps do not require any ongoing calculations or calorie counting! What? No calorie counting? Yes, because calorie counting is an archaic method that predominantly does not work. Let us reflect and learn from our past experiences as individuals, and not continue to make the same mistakes.

To set the stage for what we are going to do differently, let's highlight another ineffectual element of conventional diets. The majority tend to be of a restrictive nature, with many involving calorie counting. This compounds the restrictive eating habits set forth by the chosen diet. The traditional dogma for most diets or weight loss programs is to *eat less, exercise more*, and that calories *in* equals calories *out*, right? This means we operate at a calorie deficit. Well, how has that worked out for you, for us, or society as a whole?

We as a nation are fatter than ever before. As I already touched on, more than two-thirds of the U.S. population is currently overweight, according to the CDC. The eat less, exercise more rhetoric emphasized in dozens of popular diets (new ones pop up every year) has not proven to be a successful component of long-term health. Therefore, I would humbly submit that traditional diets and their accompanying dogma are flawed. Dieting has proven to be problematic, and ultimately does not work, in the end.

Because it is Often Viewed and Treated as Temporary

How can we bring about lasting change, or in this case, lasting weight loss, if we view dieting as temporary, or a quick fix? This is my biggest reason for not subscribing to "dieting" of any kind. I instead lean towards a more comprehensive approach, that I like to refer to as "mindful" and "intuitive" eating and behaviors. Choosing what to eat and when to eat; making better health decisions regarding sleep, stress, and exercise; while considering the associated emotional component that determines our success. Each of these are integral ingredients for reaching our overall health goals.

In order to fully experience lasting change and weight loss, you cannot simply follow a dietary regimen for a limited time, before returning to previous behaviors and expect those new results to hold long-term. No matter how much we want it, this does not happen. Most "dieting" is not designed to have long-term positive effects.

As you will now be coming to learn, many of us have fallen into the trap of yo-yo dieting, and we will discuss this more when we touch upon hormonal signals, specifically as they relate to leptin and ghrelin. These signals are an important part of the milieu (environment) that plays into our behavior. The "lack of willpower or self-control" or "lack of enough-ness," feelings that some may attribute to starting a dietary regimen, regressing, and starting over, is not as simple as these simple statements. There are actual biological, hormonal, and metabolic changes associated with dieting that can truly be an uphill battle, and may set us up for dietary failure if not understood. Remember, *You are enough* and *you are not broken.*

Of course, the goal of any diet is weight loss, right? But what if I asked you, "What is your true goal?" Is it really just to lose weight? What if I told you better health is more attainable, and weight loss comes with it? Restrictive dietary practices were never meant to be long-term behaviors. Yes, you want to fit into those favorite jeans again; yes, you want to see that long-forgotten number on the scale once again.

You are likely already envisioning the celebration party, but is this truly all you desire? Dieting is often seen as the perfect solution to short-term weight loss — let us go beyond that perception. Let us opt for the best choice, that will ultimately lead us to lasting weight loss, and a better, healthier life for the ages. Let's start strong in our method, and set the stage for *long-term* results.

When referring to healthy eating and healthy behaviors, I am often asked, "Do I have to do this forever?" Well, that depends. Do you want lasting health, energy, vitality, and to keep the weight off long-term? If your plan is to hit a certain number on the scale, finally fit back into that dress or jeans, or lose a few for an upcoming special occasion, then no, you don't have to do this forever. But if it were possible to learn that there is a way to achieve optimal health; your ideal body weight; benefit from increased energy; improved sleep; a decrease in bouts of illness; more focus, and resilience, would you be interested? If you answered "yes," keep reading.

Because it May Damage Your Metabolism

Yes, I said it. Dieting can actually be harmful to your metabolism. I am sure many of you may know someone who has personally experienced the phenomenon of yo-yo dieting. Maybe a friend, family member, or perhaps that person is even you. This is the cyclical process in which weight is lost in one dieting experience, later regained, and then struggled to be lost again. And repeat. Part of this is due to the negative psychological effects of dieting, but is it a surprise to also learn that there are negative consequences for our metabolism from dieting?

Metabolism is the sum total energy balance of all the cellular machinery and processes which are involved in creating and maintaining life and our energy levels. Despite trying your best to follow the rules designed in a particular dieting regime, have you ever experienced:

- Weight gain
- Feeling devoid of energy
- Brain fog
- Feelings of hunger to the point of incessant snacking
- A need for multiple caffeinated beverages throughout the day
- Anxiety
- That you just couldn't stop thinking of how hungry you were throughout the process?

If any of these experiences are familiar, there is a good chance your metabolism is damaged and has stopped working at peak performance and efficiency.

Yet have no fear. Just because your metabolism may have been damaged by previous behaviors, it *can* be fixed. Reversing the effects of a damaged metabolism and its functionality can become a powerful force for many attributes of a balanced life. An efficient and well-functioning metabolism is a beautiful thing indeed. It can change your life. With one, you can thrive, with elevated energy levels, increased mental clarity, focus, and alertness. An overall improved mood may also finally materialize, as you fix your metabolism.

Indeed, fixing my metabolism changed my life. The two components I focused on when carrying out this mission were the timing of my meals and the quality of my food. I eliminated the snacking. I now only eat real food, largely organic, and wild-caught or free-range well-sourced proteins. I practice intermittent fasting (time-restricted eating) for a minimum of 12 hours daily, and my exercise routine is varied, yet consistent. Whether you follow the same routine or create one of your own, I am confident these new strategies will help return you to having a high-functioning metabolism.

We now know that diets are designed for short-term "losses." But dieting long-term and bouncing between diets (yo-yo dieting) can both result in a wrecked or damaged metabolism. I have had numerous patients and others in their late 20s, 30s, and older, concerned about their state of health, come to me feeling "broken" or "falling apart." Through analysis and health history, it turned out their metabolisms were not functioning well.

Let me shout it, now, from the rooftops:

You are not broken!

There is nothing wrong with *you* as a person. However, your metabolism *may* be broken, and this can be fixed. Yes, your metabolism can be fixed.

> *You can heal.*
> *You are enough.*
> *You are worthy and capable.*
> *You've got this!*

There is a finely tuned metabolic machine our bodies rely on for balance. I have coaxed my own into gear, and have come full circle to better health. Now is the time to realize that we can thrive well into our 60s, 70s, 80s and beyond, feeling energized, focused, and full of vitality! It is not too late. You can start today!

I am now approaching fifty, and I feel more alive and vibrant than I did in my twenties! I have come to learn that this is largely due to a better functioning metabolism, and this is possible for you too! This is the very thing that fuels me to write this book. I have seen so many lives changed by caring for the metabolic functioning of our amazing human bodies. It has an exceptional capacity to truly heal and become alive again, so that you may *thrive*, not just *survive*.

Because Calorie Counting is Flawed

Spoiler Alert: 100 calories of broccoli is NOT the same as 100 calories of Oreo® cookies.

It never was, and never will be, despite what you may have learned from your favorite fitness influencer. No matter how hard we try to make them the same — equating calories eaten to calories burned during a workout — the body simply does not see them the same way.

So, why do we count calories in the first place? Fitness gurus, nutritionists, and diet influencers often seem to rely on this time-tested method of calorie counting. And why do we find it so significant? How can counting the caloric value of what we eat help us attain our fitness and weight loss goals?

Well, that's the age-old question, at least in modern dieting history. The simple answer is that it has been a common practice for at least 100 years in the mainstream nutrition space in America. However, in the scientific community, calorie counting has been around much longer than that — closer to 200 years.

Interestingly, the "science" of calorie counting, as it pertains to humans and health, is not based on human physiology, contrary to popular belief. It has been an extrapolation of a physical science principle that was never intended to be used for human health, nutrition, or physiological purposes. Yes, you heard me correctly! This supposed die-hard principle of calorie counting was never meant for nutritional use. The fact is, the first teaching of the calorie was documented in physics lectures on steam engines in the 1800s![23]

The term calorie was originally used in the English language in the 1860s, following a translation of Adolphe Ganot's French physics text *Treatise on Physics* (1863). It defined a calorie as "the heat needed to raise the temperature of one kilogram of water one degree Celsius."[23] The calorie had nothing to do with metabolism, food, or human physiology at its invention! Nothing!

In that same century, American chemist Wilbur Olin Atwater used the capitalized Calorie, or kcal that we are now familiar with, to represent one kcal on U.S. food labels as food energy.[23] The term then became commonly used after its publication in *Century* magazine, in an 1887 article. Following this, the Calorie began to enter popular American vernacular, after Atwater explained this unit in the United States Department of Agriculture (USDA) *Farmers' Bulletin* in 1894, where he provided the first U.S. food database to be used in the study of nutrition.

The Calorie, when related to human dieting and health, was further discussed in detail in what many would classify as the original bestselling book on dieting, written by Dr. Lulu Hunt Peters, entitled *Diet and Health with Key to the Calories*, published in 1918. In fact, it was through this book and Dr. Peters' many newspaper articles that she presented the concept of calorie reduction, or restriction, as the best form of weight loss. Thus, for at least 100 years, people have been attributing dieting to calorie counting.

For just a minute, let's explore the calorie counting concept. Around 1882, a device called the "bomb calorimeter" was used to determine the energy content of food, by literally burning a sample of a food, and then measuring the temperature change in the surrounding water. Yet the concept of burning food with electrical energy until final consumption or incineration, and then measuring the heat generated in its surrounding water, doesn't replicate the way food is actually metabolized in humans — not even close. Since when have we lit a fire inside our bodies, and literally burned food until it is completely transformed into ashes, carbon dioxide, and water, anyway?

This method of bomb calorimetry in the United States has been replaced by calculating energy content indirectly, by simply adding up the energy provided by the assigned energy-containing components of the basic macronutrients of food (such as protein, carbohydrates, and fats) in the so-called Modified Atwater system. This archaic technique, based largely on the experimental studies of Atwater and his colleagues from the late 1800s, is still the most common method of measuring calories today!

This is also the basis of the common technique of calculating the energy content of foods, using 4 kcal/g for carbohydrates and proteins, and 9 kcal/g for fats. This basis by which calories are measured is outdated and founded on inaccurate science. It is also not accurate to assume that all calories are created equal. For example, not all proteins and/or carbohydrates are going to represent exactly 4 kcal/g of energy. It's just not that simple!

Many other factors need to be taken into account here, not least of which is the associated fiber content of the carbohydrate food, or which amino acids are represented in the proteins, as well as the extent to which each is broken down, digested, and later absorbed and assimilated.

Let's take the case of the almond as an example of how the calories listed on food labels are often incorrect. In a 2008 study published in the *Journal of Nutrition*, U.S. Department of Agriculture researcher David Baer concluded that "Nuts are a food group for which substantial evidence suggests that the Atwater factors may be poorly predictive."[24] He found that whole almonds have about 20% less calories than the value calculated using Atwater's factors, which would typically be shown on the nutrition facts label. Two important factors not considered involve the digestion and absorption of the calories coming from whole nuts — in this case, almonds. With whole nuts, compared to nut butter or nut oils, more of the fat ends up in our stool.

Much of the fat in nuts is stored inside their cell walls, making it more of a challenge to break down during simple chewing. This causes inadequate digestion of the nut. Increased fat loss in our stool and poor digestion of the whole nut make up the 20% less calorie figure, quoted above.[24] But let us not dive too deep into the science of this. Just understand that the techniques used for measuring calories are not exact, nor are they based on actual human physiology. Until we put away this century-old method, we must relate to our food within the scope of what makes absolute and intuitive sense.

Not all calories are created equal.

Remember the opening statement? 100 calories of broccoli are not the same as 100 calories of Oreo® cookies. The obvious fact here is that an Oreo® cookie has many more ingredients (most being highly processed and even artificial) than broccoli, which has only one natural ingredient. These corresponding ingredients have a very different reaction and physiology inside our bodies, relating to which pathways and hormones are turned on or off when compared to broccoli, for example. Food is not simply its corresponding caloric value, it is *information*. In the body this information literally turns on and off genes for our benefit or detriment.

In the case of broccoli, it is mostly water, fiber, and a small number of carbs and protein. Its nutrients are vitamin C, K, iron, and potassium, and it is considered a low-calorie vegetable (about 30 calories per cup). Oreo® cookies on the other hand are full of artificial and highly processed carbohydrates (flour, sugar, and high fructose corn syrup), and are essentially devoid of any significant nutritional value, while also being calorie dense — about two cookies make up 100 calories. By comparison, it would take about 4 full cups of broccoli to make 100 calories.

So, let's compare them. Eating 4 cups of broccoli would not only give you a good source of fiber, which helps to enhance your gut health acting as a prebiotic (more on this in a later chapter), but also provide you with a great source of multiple nutrients and water, satisfying your hunger. Two cookies, however, would not likely be satiating. Rather, they would leave you hungry and craving more (from the addictive highly processed sugar, flour, and high fructose corn syrup, and corresponding dopamine rush). At the same time, they offer no significant nutritional value. Using our intuitive sense, we therefore know that broccoli is a better choice for our health.

Now, I am not begrudging you the occasional cookie. Go ahead, by all means. But are you going to eat ten or fifteen of them after you've decided to aim for optimal health? I have faith you will choose the healthier option.

One last thing — cookies will also spike your blood sugar, causing increased insulin production, which will not only make you fat, but eventually may contribute to insulin resistance, inflammation, and potential obesity and chronic disease.

Later in the book, we will further discuss the individual macronutrients such as proteins, fats, and carbohydrates, and how their interplay differs tremendously in human metabolism. You will come to see and understand that, indeed, not all calories are created equal. It *does* matter what we eat (the source and quality of our food), because food can truly be the best medicine, or a slow poison, depending on our choice. It is not simply caloric intake. Food is information that helps lead and guide trillions of processes in our amazing human body.

CHAPTER 3

Food is Medicine

> *"Let food be thy medicine*
> *and medicine be thy food."*
> -   **Hippocrates**

What You Need to Know:

- Choosing the right foods is paramount to ultimate health
- Stay away from chemically laden, industrialized processed foods (most of which come in a bag, box, or with a barcode)
- Improving your metabolism involves a diet rich in protein, healthy fats, and natural, real food carbohydrates
- Prevention of chronic diseases rests upon your decision to optimize your diet! (You can't outrun the tip of your fork)

One of the most important things I have learned in my two decades of experience as a physician is that it really does matter what we eat (not just how many calories the food we eat contains). At the end of the day, food is medicine. In fact, it is the most important and frequent medicine we can give ourselves. We have the opportunity to feed ourselves the best and most natural medicine each and every day! So, pay just as much attention to everything you eat as you would when putting medicine into your body.

Remember, food can be the most frequent and powerful medicine. It can also either be the most helpful natural medicine imaginable, or a slow poison, and *we* get to decide. It matters that much! A recent study published by *The Lancet* quantified the impact of a suboptimal diet as causing approximately 11 million deaths per year, and 255 million disability-adjusted life-years;[17] from this, one easy-to-modify risk factor alone — a poor diet!

This hits close to home for me, because I have had close family members' lives cut short in their 60s from both preventable Type 2 diabetes, heart disease and stroke complications. My own father-in-law never got to meet the majority of his grandchildren, including my two youngest children, because of his predictably premature death. It could have been delayed and even prevented had he chosen to change his diet and modify some of his behaviors. This continues to pain my wife and I: to think that it could have been different. I don't want this to happen to you or your loved ones — to have the lives of those most dear to you cut short due to risk factors and diseases that are modifiable and preventable.

JAMA estimates that more than 700,000 lives per year are lost in the United States alone, due to preventable causes of death: heart disease, stroke, and type 2 diabetes, and their associated complications.[25] Yet this does not have to be the case! Much of this prevention begins with the food we eat.

My grandmother always told me, *"You are what you eat."* And she was right! We literally use what we eat as the building blocks of our bodies. Now more than ever, it is so important to pay attention to what we put into our bodies, because there are so many harmful foods and ingredients out there; often hidden in plain sight. From pesticide-laden foods (think GMO and non-organic crops) to so many chemical-laden industrialized foods with artificial ingredients (think artificial colors, flavors, sweeteners, emulsifiers, and the dreadful vegetable or seed oils). We may even think of these processed packaged foods as staples, because that is what we may have been taught. For example: *"You need your whole grains, or low fat foods and spreads, and you should cook with vegetable oil"* and *"Breakfast is the most important meal of the day, and begins with delicious and nutritious fortified cereal."* Does this sound familiar?

Processed foods (nearly everything that comes in a package, bag or box, and with a label) should undergo additional scrutiny on our part. We will take a deep dive into this topic later in the book, but consider for now that what we eat becomes us, literally. Do you really want to be made up of Oreos,® Cheetos,® or Twinkies®?

As a physician, I would be remiss not to dive into this important and foundational topic of *food as medicine.* I will admit, this is a huge and daunting topic, and entire books have been written about it, as they should be. It is a critical and truly fundamental principle. Unfortunately, many physicians do not emphasize this simple truth enough with their patients. In fact, many individuals, both physicians and healthcare workers alike, ignore this topic altogether. But the reality and impact of this critical topic makes it vitally important to mention as we start our journey into what to eat and when to eat it. You will see that I like to focus more on what to *add*, rather than *subtract*, from our diet, as there is so much more that is healthy and simultaneously delicious that can add to both our enjoyment of food as well as adding important nutrients that our bodies both need and desire. And the basic foods or what I affectionately call the "food-like substances" to avoid can be summarized in a couple simple rules which will be explained shortly.

Anything and everything we consume, food or drink, is not simply calories generated after being incinerated in a calorimeter, but instead detailed information and instructions to our body on both what to do and how to do it. Food is involved in directing the expression of our genes. The very food we eat dictates which genes get turned on or off, plays a role in gene expression, and to a large extent can cause or contribute to health or disease. It is that simple, yet profoundly impactful. We will get into this a little more later in the book as we talk about epigenetics. For now, let's remember that food is the most powerful and frequent medicine we can take, so we should pay attention to what we eat!

A clear example of a case when food was not recognized as medicine was what I witnessed in my medical training at a world-renowned children's hospital in California a couple of decades ago. I kid you not, this reputable healthcare institution had a McDonald's® restaurant on the first floor, inside the hospital! In fact, I witnessed many instances of physicians encouraging families to bring their ailing hospital and clinic patients this SAD food, which may have not only helped cause or contribute to their ailments, but was likely making them worse. From oncologists to pediatricians and other specialists, it was almost criminal to witness this absurdity. Unfortunately, this business flourished for over twenty years in one of the most medically advanced hospitals in the world. Somehow it was forgotten that food is medicine.

Everything we put into our bodies produces some effect — good, bad, or otherwise. To overlook this makes no sense and is, quite frankly, ignorant. One cannot put substances into their body and believe with certainty that this consumption will not produce some effect. Not only are we made of what we eat, but basic laws of physiology and physics preclude the notion of a zero effect from what we eat or drink. Though I am sure there are times we would hope and wish that what we put into our bodies did not matter or affect us in any way, this is not reality. Our life instead depends on these choices. It is that simple!

I have found this primordial truth to often be unrecognized and underappreciated. For example, a T-shirt I saw the other day had a picture of a raccoon in gym clothes doing a massive deadlift, and with the bar bending it stated, "I work out so I can eat garbage." This has become a sad truth. Even worse, it has become the popular opinion of many fitness influencers, trainers, and many of my physician colleagues.

It is not entirely their fault. Data suggests that medical schools, in their typical four years of curriculum, inadequately teach future doctors about nutrition.26 Out of thousands of training hours, only twenty-four hours (one or two classes) are dedicated to nutrition instruction. Only 30% of over one hundred medical schools surveyed in this study had a formal nutrition class requirement for graduating at all. This under-training of physicians in nutrition is part of the problem. At the same time, knowledge within the lay public is similarly wanting.

The underlying dogma is that it does not matter much what you eat, as long as you exercise, right? Calories in equals calories out? Wrong! You cannot simply exercise away all the ill effects of a bad diet, it is just not possible (think of the broccoli versus Oreo® example). *No* amount of exercise will *ever* cancel out the effects of a poor diet — none! (Read that again.)

Moreover, what we choose to consume may actually be the single most important act to lead us on a path towards optimal health and wellness, or chronic disease. It is largely our choice, and within our control, which path we take. We've got this!

To bring to light the magnitude of this concept, according to the CDC, as much as 40% of the annual deaths in the United States from each of the five leading causes are entirely preventable. This means in the U.S. alone up to 360,000 deaths per year could be entirely prevented by an improved diet and better lifestyle choices.[27] Worldwide, seven of the top ten leading causes of death are non-communicable, largely modifiable, and preventable.[17] Heart disease is considered the most common cause of death worldwide both in women and men. It is, to a great extent, a preventable and modifiable disease, while it accounted for approximately 17.9 million deaths annually worldwide. Sadly, that number has been climbing each year, per the World Health Organization (WHO).[210]

Type 2 diabetes (essentially entirely preventable) is now among the top ten causes of death worldwide, and is responsible for the largest rise in male deaths, with an 80% increase since the year 2000.[17] Noncommunicable diseases (non-infectious) accounted for 74% of deaths globally in 2019. This number is not only staggering, but for me as a physician, entirely frustrating, as the majority of the top ten causes of death are to a large degree preventable, and have their problematic roots in diet and lifestyle, not genetics.

Why do we then, as a nation and a world, not focus on responding to these numbers through the lens of easily modifiable risk factors — diet and lifestyle? Instead, we spend billions of dollars on temporizing pharmaceutical treatments, while ignoring the underlying root causes. Recognizing and treating food as medicine is paramount in changing this.

The mortality rates from heart disease and stroke are ridiculously high, significantly affecting our economy. More than 868,000 Americans die of heart disease or stroke every year — that is more than one-third of all deaths. There is a minimum cost to our healthcare system of $214 billion per year, as well as an additional $138 billion in lost work productivity! Diabetes and obesity are also high on the list, costing $327 billion and $147 billion each year, respectively.[28]

Together, these preventable diseases run a tab of nearly a trillion dollars annually in the U.S. alone. This is a staggering revelation that underlines how preventable these diseases can be through diet and lifestyle modification. This is why I wrote this book! We can do better on a global, national, and individual level. I humbly submit that by doing so, we will improve our lives significantly, positively impacting the national and global health care system, and our personal bottom line.

Beyond the numerous chemical therapeutics (pharmaceutical medications) people take to combat chronic disease, I would humbly submit that the foods and drinks we consume are just as important, if not more so, in the grand scheme of better health. I can say that, in my two decades-plus experience in medicine, the majority of the medications I have seen prescribed for the most common health ailments (diabetes, heart disease, hypertension, stroke, and mood disorders such as stress, anxiety, and depression) could largely be replaced by treating food as the medicinal remedy. Thus, optimizing one's health from a dietary perspective can be a profound lever in making this drastically needed change.

What is interesting to me is that many people, including physicians, may think this approach is controversial — prescribing diet and lifestyle modifications over pharmaceuticals — despite overwhelming support from a multitude of studies and research. Diet and lifestyle modification addresses chronic ailments from the root — the preferred method of improving lives for long-term wellness.

The need for the majority of type 2 diabetes medications, for example, could be avoided by altering one's dietary and lifestyle habits, which would in turn optimize weight, thereby tackling insulin sensitivity. This is talked about at length in the phenomenal book, *Why We Get Sick*, by Dr. Benjamin Bikman, whom I had the pleasure of interviewing on my podcast *Unshakeable Health*. Other excellent books have also been written on this subject, like Dr. William Li's *Eat to Beat Disease* (also a podcast guest), so I will not belabor the point here. But for a more in-depth understanding of diet and its correlation to improved health, I highly recommend reading each of these powerful books.

However, it is important to still discuss the concept and thought process behind this here, how we can apply it, and by doing so, how this will allow us to better care for our bodies physically, mentally, and emotionally.

Since our body does not operate in a vacuum and is greatly influenced by what we put in it, I will focus a measurable amount of space on our metabolism, and its corresponding fuels, in the chapters to come. The food, or fuel, discussed is composed of the major macronutrients: protein, fats, and carbohydrates. We will focus not only on *what* to eat, but what *not* to, and *when*, in order to fuel our bodies with what will help fix our metabolism and power it best.

The prevention of chronic diseases and ailments is directly related to dietary choices. Poor dietary choices are directly related to metabolic health. Therefore, improving metabolic health is one way to change disease from the root.

Before rolling up our sleeves and diving into metabolism, let us first focus on *what* and *when* we should eat, and a few ways to look at weight management.

Let's go!

When You Eat Matters as Much as *What* You Eat: Intermittent Fasting Made Easy

---

What You Need to Know:

- Incorporating intermittent fasting into your dietary routine opens a natural pathway to a healthier metabolism and gut
- Try the "CIRCADIAN FAST," which is simply an overnight fast plus a couple hours on either end, or eating during an 8-12 hour window and fasting for the remaining 12–16 hours
- Break the cycle of a "traditional" carb-filled breakfast by starting the day with healthy proteins and fat, fresh fruit, and yogurt, for example
- Practice mindful eating, and your mental, emotional, and physical acuity will become your new high

---

Is intermittent fasting or time-restricted eating worthy of the recent hype? My humble opinion is a resounding YES. This is not because a celebrity or social media CEO may have done it and then tweeted about it. Nor because longevity expert Dr. David Sinclair does it. Instead, intermittent fasting is a tried and true health practice that has been safely and successfully used by humans for millennia. Our bodies are literally designed for this!

Looking to our past does not make it difficult to appreciate the roots of this beneficial ancient practice. It was normal human behavior for our hunter-gatherer ancestors, as well as those that followed them. It was even a common practice a hundred years ago, in its simplest form — what I like to call circadian fasting. I even practiced it throughout my youth, though I didn't know it, for we did not have a name for it back then.

Fasting, in one form or another, has been used by nearly every culture, and every religion, for millennia. It all likely began as a way to survive, and was later practiced for its physical, mental, and spiritual health benefits. In fact, Paracelsus, a physician and philosopher in the early 1500s, is credited with saying, "Fasting is the greatest remedy — the physician within." He was right. Fasting promotes health and healing in a myriad of ways.

Our hunter-gatherer ancestors and even those living only 100 years ago did not generally have 24-hour access to food as we do today. Yes, they could hunt and gather for hours, but there was no reliable system of regulated storage. Today, when we want milk we simply walk to our refrigerator and pour a glass. Yet our ancestors could only consume milk within a few minutes of milking the cow. With no refrigeration, milking enough to last a week was not an option. Hunting and gathering berries, fish, meats, tubers, and crops from the land each day was performed on the basis of immediate need.

This consistently led to hours out of the day when those ancestors did not eat: averaging 12–16 hours, perhaps more, when they were either sleeping or working to obtain their food. We also have the same DNA and metabolic machinery capable of this moderate fasting interval, and it is significantly healthy and beneficial to do so. Its rewards are not limited only to the moment (most people will notice an increase in energy and a sharpened mental focus which likely helped greatly in daily hunts on which our ancestors regularly embarked) but also has significant long-term, health-promoting effects: from improved metabolic health to increased longevity.

Though I was unaware of it as a child, we, and many families during that time (in the 70s and early 80s), practiced time-restricted feeding, a common type of intermittent fasting. We did not have a name for it back then, nor did we realize that we were doing it. Let me explain. We would normally eat dinner at about 5 P.M. each day, and were nearly always done by 6 P.M. Then the "kitchen was closed," by decree of my mother, and we did not eat again until about 7:30 A.M. the following day. We definitely did not do "midnight snacks" at our house. Thus, we had a circadian fasting window of 12–14 hours daily, without even knowing it!

And guess what? We survived, and did not suffer any untoward effects! Back then, none of our family of eight developed obesity or type 2 Diabetes, which is now sadly rising rapidly in children, youth, and adults worldwide. In our house, we simply did not know of life any other way. It was our normal routine, and trust me, we did not go hungry.

For our hunter-gatherer ancestors, this was likely a bit more extreme, as it may have taken several hours to either find or hunt their food. Likely, their overnight fasting window may have been closer to 14–18 hours, but I think you see the point. Fasting has been part of our history for millennia, until the modern-day inventions of snack foods, 24-hour availability of drive-thrus, supermarkets, and of course the readily accessible pantry and refrigerator.

Indeed, my family unknowingly practicing intermittent fasting (time-restricted feeding) led to our decent health, where neither my parents, nor siblings, nor I, were overweight as children, adolescents, and into early adulthood. This is not to brag or overstate this memory of mine, but to instead substantiate a realization of how a simple everyday practice contributed to our health and vitality for many years. While I wish I could say that none of us in my family have ever struggled with weight, that is not the case.

Times changed, years passed, and we grew up. My parents got older and most of my family (myself included) made some unhealthy modifications to the circadian fasting we grew up practicing. The common practice of snacking and eating late meals, followed by early breakfasts with readily available SAD (Standard American Diet) breakfast staples: cold cereals, bagels, croissants, and scones, crept in.

Our collective health declined. Some of us did circle back to the circadian fasting of our upbringing, though other pressures of daily life, modern conveniences, and social acceptance of new societal norms have caused several in my family to struggle with obesity, type 2 diabetes and insulin resistance.

My greatest hope is that we will all find some collective value in this age-old practice, that carries one of the biggest "bangs" for our buck in improved health, weight loss, and longevity. In fact, beyond its tried and true nature, it is one of the simplest weight loss and health strategies to embrace and incorporate into your life long-term; and it's totally FREE!

In subsequent chapters, we will discuss the importance and benefits of daytime light exposure, and evening blue light avoidance to optimize sleep, by mimicking the natural circadian clock of our ancestors. Yet for now, we will touch upon the second major factor for optimized circadian function, which acts as a helpful adjuvant to light exposure — *the timing of our food*. I have found that this is just as important as *what* we choose to eat. Timing matters, period.

Early studies of this principle, as reported in the scientific journal *Cell Metabolism* in 2012, showed this very concept in action. Dr. Sachidananda Panda and colleagues at the Salk Institute in La Jolla, California studied two groups of identical mice, who were fed identical diets with the same amount of calories. The two groups had very different outcomes, based only on the difference in the timing of the intake.[29]

Interestingly, both groups in each case were fed the same diet, composed of the same foods and quantities of food (they also redid the trial using different types of diets, with different macronutrients holding it constant between the two groups), with the same amount of total calories. However, one group had access to food anytime (could eat or snack *ad lib*), whereas the other group had access to the same food and same calories only during an 8-hour feeding window, while the remaining 16 hours were spent fasting (no caloric intake).

The difference was literally night and day! The group that was able to eat *ad lib* not only got fatter but also showed signs of significant metabolic damage, including insulin resistance, fatty liver, and inflammation, as well as an impaired lipid metabolism.[29] On the other hand, the other group that practiced time-restricted eating did not get fat (was 28% lighter), had improved metabolic parameters (better lipid and glucose metabolism with less insulin resistance and a healthier liver), as well as decreased inflammation. Time-restricted feeding for the win!

This was one of the first of many studies to show the tremendous benefits of intermittent fasting and time-restricted feeding. So what exactly is this, anyway? It's super simple, and we all likely do some version of it already. Intermittent fasting (IF) is a general term that refers to cycles of fasting and eating.

A popular variety of intermittent fasting known as TRF (Time-Restricted Feeding) is the 16/8 method — where one eats during an 8-hour window and fasts for the remaining 16 hours. Say you skip breakfast and eat your first meal at noon or 12 P.M., then you would stop eating after dinner, or 8 P.M., repeating that schedule the following day by eating your first meal at 12 P.M. This may be a little much for those just starting, but it gives you an idea.

Most of us already fast eight or more hours a day, typically while we sleep. What I recommend is trying to extend this window a little at a time, to eventually be able to fast somewhere between 12–16 hours a couple of days a week. This is what I like to call a "circadian fast" (as it is something we have done for millennia and is consistent with our ideal circadian rhythm). It seems the "magic" happens somewhere around the 12 to 13-hour mark. While more on this will be covered later, for now make this your benchmark for success.

Another common type of intermittent fast is the 5:2 method. You pick 2 out of the 7 days of the week (not necessarily consecutive) to minimize your calories, usually keeping them around 500–600 Calories each of the two days. The remaining 5 days you continue to eat your normal amount of healthy calories.

Another type of fast is the 24-hour fast. This can be done 1–2 times a month. It can be done after dinner, say starting at 7 P.M., then fasting 24 hours until dinner the next day at 7 P.M.

As you can see, there are many variations. I personally do a circadian fast about 5 days a week, and shoot for it to last between 14-16 hours on average. I also incorporate a 24-hour fast about once a month, depending on my needs and schedule. I have found this fast to be especially rejuvenating, as I don't have to worry at all about food for a full 24 hours (you can drink water or zero-calorie fluids/tea/coffee during this time to stay well hydrated). This time, free of the concerns related to food (the prep, shopping, eating, cleanup, etc.), really helps me mentally sharpen my focus, spikes my creativity, and is often one of the more memorable days of the month.

One of the things I love most about the time-restricted feeding model is that it is simple to do and does not require any extra planning or grocery shopping. It actually simplifies things! However, I have also noticed, both with myself and many others while practicing any variation of intermittent fasting, that, if we don't mix it up sometimes, the body tends to adapt to its new fasting format, and things stall. The weight loss benefits, for example, may plateau.

A friend of mine started the circadian fast technique on my recommendation, and after a few weeks had adjusted to the 16/8 variation. She did this daily for 2 months, and lost 25 pounds, before reaching a stalling point where no further weight was lost despite keeping her 16/8 windows intact (her goal was 30 pounds). She even started to gain a little weight back. She had not noticeably changed what she was eating, the quantity, or the timing. What was likely happening was that her metabolism had "adapted" to this new 16/8 program, and started to conserve energy (calories) for the 16 hours daily she was fasting (her metabolic rate slowed), and she went into conservation mode.

This is called "metabolic adaptation." This occurs due to a combination of metabolic slowing, with changes in hunger and satiety hormones.[30, 31] At this point, I recommended she take 2 days off each week, without imposing strict windows (where she did not necessarily change what she was eating). Taking a break on the 16-hour fast two or three days a week, and continuing to eat real whole foods, allowed her to lose those last stubborn 5 pounds!

She also told me that she was feeling more energetic, lively, mentally focused and clear, less inflamed (swollen), had less joint pains, and had a much simpler and less stressful life. She was mostly eating two meals per day, and was saving a lot of time preparing, cooking, eating, and cleaning up, so she was free to pursue the things she truly enjoyed. It was a win-win!

This metabolic adaptation is a product of our ancestry, and was literally what kept our predecessors alive during times of famine. We have also preserved these same genes, and our body can switch them on if it is faced with fasting or caloric restriction on a regular basis. This was a huge advantage when food was scarce.

Our present environment, with 24-hour access to food, however, is a recipe for weight gain, unless we learn how to optimize metabolic adaptation. This can easily be done by eating natural, real whole foods, and incorporating the activity of fasting in a varied routine, to prevent the body from adapting by conserving calories and slowing down metabolism.

This is a practice that, like many others I describe in the book, is best when individualized to your specific needs. Please also remember to discuss this practice or any changes to your dietary or health routine with your healthcare provider first so that it can be tailored to your individual needs. When that magic happens for you, you will see the many powerful benefits of this age-old practice.

When I became aware of the tremendous benefits of IF a few years ago, I sat back and reflected upon my own patterns and behaviors around hunger and eating. It was hard to break up with the traditional belief that "breakfast is the most important meal of the day," so I continued eating my morning meals anyway. In 2011, Kamada and colleagues investigated the "WHAT" regarding breakfast, in a study published in the journal *Gastroenterology and Hepatology from Bed to Bench*.

They concluded from their research that "the types and quality of breakfast [are] key as regular breakfast consumption alone did not show adequate health benefits."[32] They also found that lower glycemic load (GL) foods (generally those unprocessed or minimally processed), and higher protein intake at breakfast were found to be associated with higher energy levels. In other words, what matters more than whether breakfast is the most important meal or not is *what* you are eating at breakfast. In addition, we also now know that the timing is of tremendous significance, too.

Whatever the importance you apply to breakfast, just remember that *you* get to decide what you put in your mouth! I personally love my breakfast, though I tend to eat it sometime between 10 A.M. and 1 P.M., depending on the day. I follow the "pack it with powerful protein" mantra, by eating several eggs and Greek yogurt. I avoid most carbohydrates at breakfast (bread, bagels, donuts, croissants, scones, pancakes and even the majority breakfast cereals unless it is a drizzle of grain-free granola atop of my yogurt), and may also add some seasonal berries to my Greek yogurt at the end of the meal.

When I listen to my body by practicing mindful or intuitive eating, I generally do not feel like eating until I have been up for a couple of hours anyway. Though as I have experimented with this practice of time-restricted eating I have found that I benefit even more from advancing ahead my window (eating breakfast earlier nowadays) and also ending my window with an earlier dinner, or sometimes even skipping dinner altogether depending on what my body dictates. Though I still shoot for a minimum of 12 hours between dinner and breakfast, I allow my body to dictate when to eat and try to be more mindful and intuitive rather than following a strict hourly routine.

I have also found in my work with many people who have also incorporated this practice that there is no exact one size fits all approach (You will see this is a common theme in the book that each practice needs to be personalized and adapted to the individual. This individualized approach is often called precision medicine – which I feel is also the *best* medicine).

With respect to intermittent fasting I have seen in my experience that women and men, for example, can have very different needs and ways in which to best adapt this tool to their individual circumstances. For example, for menstruating women, I would not recommend pushing the fasting window mid cycle near ovulation nor at the end of the month when they are premenstrual as these are times where their bodies tend to benefit from increased calories and less lengthy fasting windows. However, in the week just after menses, or at the beginning of their cycle, many women find that they can easily add hours to their fasting window without much difficulty. Once again, please be mindful and listen to your body and your needs and find out what works best for you.

In addition, I have found that when I submit to this age-old practice, the fasting hours are among the most energizing, invigorating, creative, and productive hours of my day — my mind feels sharp and focused, and my body is ready to "crush it." This often means I take advantage of this energy and vitality, and do my morning "hunt" (an exercise routine, choosing between surfing, skiing, snowboarding, biking, resistance training, and walking — I have a newfound LOVE for walking).

Intermittent fasting is also akin to a daily housekeeping service for our body that can clean, refresh, and invigorate our body systems so that they run smoother, stronger, more efficiently, and become less prone to disease and infection. If we do not have an active plan for keeping our bodies in optimal health, we lose out on the process that enables us to reach prime, long-term health.

Our bodies are our temples. Therefore, regular housekeeping is necessary to maintain its optimal working condition for the duration. Enter *autophagy*, which plays a vital role in accomplishing this task. The term means "self-eating," which is the body's way of doing its own internal housekeeping, by clearing out old damaged cells or proteins in order to regenerate newer healthier ones in their place while also disposing of the waste or toxins that build up during the ongoing process of metabolism. This process of autophagy is the one by which our body renews and regenerates, and can do so on a daily basis if we allow for it to take place.

Autophagy primarily occurs while we are fasting (or not eating).[33] For us, this can happen at night while we are sleeping, and extend into the day if we continue our fast. If we add 2–6 hours to this window, say 2–3 hours after dinner and then 2–3 hours after waking, before we consume anything with calories, we are off to a great start for our time-restricted feeding style of intermittent fasting.

Drinking water, as well as natural beverages without calories (organic tea or unsweetened coffee), is fine during fasting windows. Keeping calories low or preferably at zero during the fasting window is ideal, because calories stop the fast (especially if there are any carbohydrates present in the food) as they cause insulin to rise, which shuts down the fat-burning stage your body is in during intermittent fasting.

But what about drinks with artificial sweeteners like zero-calorie soda or drinks with Nutrasweet, Splenda, and the like? Avoid them like the plague! Besides the toxic chemical nature of these artificial sweeteners, they may be linked to increases in metabolic disease and obesity. They are also harmful to the health of your gut (more on this later).34

If you are doing a prolonged occasional fast, say 24–48 hours, drinking water and electrolytes is recommended, as well as medical supervision. Prolonged fasts, though I don't recommend them too often, have shown to be especially useful for autophagy. As I mentioned, I personally do one 24-hour fast a month on a regular basis. If this is your preferred model, start with the 24-hour fast, rather than the 48-hour; it is less intense as it only involves skipping two meals.

In December of 2019, Dr. Mark Mattson from Johns Hopkins Neurosciences and Dr. Rafael de Cabo wrote a great review article in the prestigious *New England Journal of Medicine*, which detailed some of the major benefits and physiologic effects of intermittent fasting. It is well done, illustrative, and easy to follow, and I would highly recommend reading it. Some major benefits included: decreased obesity and Type 2 diabetes, less insulin resistance, less heart disease, less cancer and neurodegenerative disease, better lipid profiles, improved metabolic health (especially in those mighty mitochondria), and a decrease in the inflammatory or autoimmune illnesses.[35]

Improved gut health is another significant benefit recently discovered with regards to the type of time-restricted feeding I practice. Specifically, the beneficial intestinal bacteria *Akkermansia muciniphila* and *Bacteroides fragilis* have increased abundance when fasting 12–18 hours, as is practiced during the holy month of Ramadan.[36] If that was not enough, a recently released study in *Behavioural Brain Research* from April 2021 suggested that intermittent fasting also promotes anxiolysis (less anxiety).[37] New studies are being released all the time on numerous benefits of intermittent fasting, but do you want to know why I like it best? Yes, the benefits are amazing, read on.

The thing I like most of all about intermittent fasting is the ease and simplicity of putting it into practice. It does not require a notebook, a calorie counting app, new foods, or any sophisticated equipment whatsoever. It only requires a clock. It does not necessarily require any changes to the food you eat or quantity, making it easy to maintain for both the short and long-term!

You can start wherever you are comfortable, and slowly increase the fasting window until you reach your desired goal of somewhere between 12–16 hours. I usually shoot for 14, but sometimes I go 16, 18, or as little as 12 hours. You can be flexible, and should be! Let's say you have friends or family in town, and they want to have brunch with you at 10 A.M., yet you normally don't eat your first meal until 12 or 1 P.M. That's totally fine — you can adjust it, and eat with them!

In addition, I have found that not only is it a simple and relatively easy practice to add to my healthy lifestyle, but it also gives me more time to focus on other important life matters, as typically I have less meals to plan and shop for, prepare, and then eat — giving me several hours more time each and every week!

In the case that you may have started fasting for the first time, and normally your overnight (circadian) fast is only the 8 or 9 hours you sleep, this is totally fine! You could start by adding thirty minutes to an hour onto your overnight fast, to either side of your sleeping window (whichever is easier in order to start with a WIN), and then lengthen this by 30–60 minutes each week as you get used to it. You could be up to a 12-hour overnight fast in as little as one month!

You can also go either faster or slower, depending on how you are feeling. Remember, there is no right or wrong pace. Take your time, listen to your body, and I think you will be pleasantly surprised with the ease, simplicity, and huge benefits. (Please always consult with your doctor or qualified healthcare provider when you embark on any new dietary or health practice.)

So then — simplicity, tremendous benefits, and it's absolutely FREE! It's a win-win-win! This is a trifecta I can totally subscribe to! I hope you'll now also see the power of intermittent fasting — an age-old yet extremely powerful technique! Remember, just listen to your body, and adjust as you are comfortable. You've got this!

Just wait until you read about how water can benefit your waistline too! And keep in mind, drinking water is ALWAYS allowed during whichever intermittent fasting type you try, as you should want, and need, to keep your body hydrated. Read on to see why!

Water Can Help You Lose Weight

What You Need to Know:

- Water is essential, natural, and healthy. Drink until your heart's content
- All on its own, water can boost your metabolic rate, which helps burn calories
- Remaining properly hydrated can also help to decrease cravings for unhealthy snacks
- If you drink 2–3 liters of water/fluids daily, this is a very good place to start

---

Have you heard of the phenomenon of water-induced thermogenesis? If not, you won't want to miss this. Water-induced thermogenesis has been shown to be a free and easy mechanism to not only help with hydration and satiety, but also boost metabolism and even help you lose weight. Who doesn't like the sound of that? Can the simple act of drinking water and staying hydrated help you lose weight? Yes!

Importantly, it does so in several ways. First, drinking water has been shown to actually trigger a boost in metabolic rate all by itself — water alone can boost your metabolism! This was explained in a 2003 study reported in the *Journal of Clinical Endocrinology and Metabolism,* which showed that simply drinking a half liter of water (about sixteen ounces) can increase your metabolic rate by as much as 30%.[38]

This can then generate energy to the tune of about 100kJ (Kilojoules). So, if you drink sixteen ounces of water four times a day, your body can create up to 400kJ EXTRA of metabolic energy — daily! This energy can help to burn fat if you are (as the name suggests) in fat-burning mode — see the later chapter on metabolism — or by burning excess carbohydrates.

Yes, drinking water can help you lose weight by increasing your metabolic rate, and burning more calories. But the weight loss benefits of water do not end here. If you drink water before each meal (sixteen ounces, three times a day, thirty minutes before the meal), you can also increase your satiety for the upcoming meal. You likely will eat less food, and consume fewer calories during the meal, creating space to potentially lose weight.

In addition to the thermogenic effect of water, and its bonus utility of helping with satiety for meals, staying properly hydrated can also help with your cravings and overall health! I have seen this quite often in my practice — simply drinking a glass of water between meals when one feels lower energy or hunger can oftentimes curb those sensations, helping with overall hydration and weight loss simultaneously.

You may even get the same satisfaction from a glass of water as you would from a snack. Think about this next time you feel the urge to snack between meals. Drink a full glass of water instead. Better yet, consider water with electrolytes. Make sure to steer away from most sports drinks, though, as they typically contain sugar and unhealthy sweeteners. As you will read in the metabolism chapter, drinking sugary drinks elevates your glucose and insulin — kicking you out of fat-burning mode.

If we are dehydrated, and especially if we are low on electrolytes, we will often crave salt or salty things, leading to snacking. Hey, we all love potato chips. But let's be honest — it's what's available, easy to grab, and yummy! When was the last time you consumed a pinch of sea salt when you craved something salty? Doesn't seem likely to happen, does it? But it could, if we ditch the chips at the supermarket and they never make it into our pantry in the first place. Out of sight, out of mind, right?

The good news: salt cravings may dissipate if we hydrate with water and add electrolytes — rather than snacking! These cravings may subside when drinking water (with or without electrolytes). Genius!

This is because both hunger and thirst are regulated by the same part of the brain, the hypothalamus. So, are those signals getting crossed, or misinterpreted? This often happens — when we are actually thirsty, we may get the signal that we are hungry — and simply drinking six to eight ounces of water can curtail this in a hurry. So, next time you feel a little bit hungry between meals, instead of reaching for a snack, try drinking eight ounces of water and see if that does the trick. Deal?

So, why not name a few of these benefits of water and hydration, to really highlight my point? Well, drinking water and staying hydrated can help with both physical and mental performance, brain health, mental acuity, sharpness, and sleep, while also reducing constipation, to name but a few. Water can also help prevent kidney stones (a super debilitating and painful condition when you have it), prevent headaches, and much more!

In fact, an important meta-analysis in 2018 from the journal *Medicine & Science in Sports & Exercise* further elucidated the importance of hydration on brain performance.[39] It showed that if one is as little as two percent dehydrated, this can have a significant impact on cognitive performance, attention, executive function, and motor coordination. So, why wouldn't you want to stay hydrated? It is an inexpensive weight management system, with tremendous benefits to your overall health.

Now, how much do we need to drink to stay appropriately hydrated? Well, that depends on the individual, but a good baseline rule of thumb is to drink half of your body weight, in pounds, in the ounces of water you consume a day. So, according to this rule, someone who weighs 150 pounds would start by drinking 75 ounces of water a day for baseline needs.

According to the journal *Nutrition Reviews*, a daily water intake of 3.7L for adult men and 2.7L for adult women should meet the needs of the vast majority of people.[40] Strenuous physical exercise and heat stress can greatly increase daily water needs, and the individual variability between people can be substantial.

So, the exact quantity one should drink daily is typically between two and three liters, and will vary based upon the individual, local circumstances (whether you live in the humid south or dry cool tundra, for example), as well as their level of activity. An easy rule of thumb is to monitor the color of your urine to see how you are doing with hydration. The goal is to basically have clear-looking urine, light yellow or similar to the color of water. If it is more yellow, or a darker yellow, this is typically a sign of potential dehydration. Personally, I aim to drink between two and three liters of water or fluid a day, which is (70–102 ounces — I weigh 150 pounds). As well as this, I check my urine color and my activity level, to gauge how much I am sweating.

What I have also learned in my twenty years of experience as a physician is that most of us experience chronically mild dehydration on a daily basis, simply because we do not drink adequate amounts of water. A good way to keep track is to buy a BPA-free glass or aluminum water bottle, and calculate how many times you'd need to fill it daily to maintain your 70–100 ounces or so. It seems like a lot at first, but when you include the sixteen ounces of water before each meal, and sipping on it every time you feel hungry, it is actually quite easy to accomplish. It may truly be a game-changer for you! Just what the doctor ordered — clear, pure, refreshing H_2O!

> *I have been pleasantly surprised over the years by how simple, yet powerful, this hydration effect can be, and have witnessed thousands of people improve both their health and waistline by smarter incorporation of water into their daily routine.*

So, here's to a successful daily water routine. Cheers!

Our Mighty Metabolism

What You Need to Know:

- Our metabolism **does not** slow down with age until at least the age of 60
- A healthy metabolism plays a pivotal role in your energy levels and managing weight loss and gain
- **What** we eat truly affects our metabolism
- Optimizing our metabolism requires an active lifestyle and a balanced, healthy diet (remember: real and whole food, fruits, veggies, plenty of water, and exercise!)
- Ketones and healthy fats are great alternative fuels for maintaining metabolic health

---

Have you ever said to yourself, "I wish I had the metabolism of so-and-so. You know, that person who is thin, fit, and can eat whatever they want, never gaining any weight?" If so, you are not alone.

Indeed, your metabolism matters. It is part and parcel of our everyday noticeable health, energy levels, and managing weight loss or gain. Unfortunately, this is another one of those misunderstood topics in the traditional medicine and commonplace health and fitness space. Regarding our understanding of metabolism, their delivery of inaccurate messages has often led us as a society down the wrong path.

My experience has been that medical, health, and fitness teachings have not delved into far enough detail regarding how *what* we eat truly affects us in terms of our metabolism. It definitely matters! Instead, the focus too often has erroneously been *"calories in equals calories out,"* or *"eat less, exercise more,"* without much emphasis placed on *what* exactly we should eat. At times, when the discussion reels around to what or when to eat, it is often flat-out wrong. What we consume for fuel through food and drink and for sustenance *does* actually make a difference towards our overall health.

What we digest does not find its way into a vacuum, black hole, or the proverbial "bottomless pit" I was accused of having as a teenager because of my voracious appetite. As discussed in the chapter *Food is Medicine*, what we put into our bodies has a significant effect on our health, and in this case, our metabolism. In fact, what we eat in large part affects, and ultimately makes up, our metabolism. No two people are the same, as indeed no two people will eat exactly the same things. Therefore, no two people will have exactly the same metabolism. This is a fascinating concept we will dig into later.

I will use an engine metaphor to help shed light on metabolism, to help conceptualize this point. In order to get our engine (metabolism) running smoothly without "throwing a rod," rattling, or stalling — so it "purrs" or runs smoothly and effortlessly — the type of fuel we put into it makes a huge difference. Not only are we what we eat, but we are also what our food has eaten, or been fed and grown with, as well. This is why seeking out well-sourced, high-quality foods is so important for our health.

In essence, what we eat actually becomes us! Paying attention to what you eat, where it comes from, and how much of it you eat, is paramount to metabolic health. We can positively change our metabolism by being mindful of what affects it and how it functions. What leads us towards health or illness is not based so much on age, inheritance, or genetics, but *how* we treat and take care of what we've got!

The different types of calories we consume — the source and quality of them — allow our cellular engine to either operate at ideal efficiency and flexibility, or not. Furthermore, the fuel we ingest breaks down into three basic macronutrients: carbohydrates, proteins, and fat, and we will cover each of these in detail in the coming chapters.

Yes, we may look to people who are thin or appear healthy, and who may seem to have a lot of energy, and say, "I want their metabolism," or, "I bet they have a faster metabolism than I do." But let us look at this another way. The notion of a fast or slow metabolism does not actually exist in the way it has often been reported.

It ultimately comes down to whether or not we have a finely tuned or unbroken metabolism. And much of the difference generally stems from what our engines are fed. Each person feeds or treats his or her metabolism differently. Therefore, how one's metabolism behaves from one person to the next also varies.

Another very common misplaced belief that many of us may hold is that metabolism slows down as we age. Well, this is not exactly true. Our metabolism, in and of itself, does not slow down significantly with age, necessarily. Rather, *we* do. What changes for us as adults, *is* us. We change, not so much our metabolism.

Let me give you an example — have you ever watched children play? Kids and youths traditionally spend lots of time playing, running, chasing, and being active, right? If any of you had to follow my kids around for a day, it would exhaust you, as they seem to have nonstop energy! Yet as we age, our metabolism does not necessarily slow down by itself. What actually happens is *we* slow down, generally becoming more sedentary. Yet many of us, including me, would argue that we are just as active as we were in our 20s. Whatever the case, I would venture to say that most adults decrease their physical activity as they age, putting on a few extra pounds, which further guarantees that they will slow down.

As a result of decreased activity, we may also lose muscle mass, which, as we will find out soon, is key to maintaining a healthy metabolic rate. In a landmark study reported in the journal *Science* in August 2021, the authors reported that metabolism in adults, or their total daily energy expenditure, was actually stable from 20–60 years of age![41] Here, the notion that our metabolism does not slow down as adults, at least between the ages of 20–60 years, is validated.

Nowadays many adults, and our children, spend a lot of time interacting with our phones and other devices. We don't move enough, and certainly not as much as we did in our youth (the pre-device era). Coupled with the Standard American Diet, this stands as a recipe for obesity and type 2 diabetes, both of which have rapidly increased in children and adults in recent years. After sixty years of age, the data for the effects on adult metabolism is less clear, but on average, the rate of energy expenditure seems to decline along with muscle mass. Fortunately, this does not have to be the case.

Knowing that we can have the same metabolism we did when we were twenty, at least until we are sixty, is empowering. This means that we *can* do something to maintain our metabolic health, in order to reach our goal of overall long-term health. I recommend we focus on what we *can* control (movement, diet, and other healthy habits such as sleep and stress optimization). And whether we have reached the awesome age of sixty or not, being mindful of what we put into our mouths, how much and when, and being active on a regular and consistent basis, are important ways to keep our engines purring. Yes, we can positively change our metabolism! The ball is definitely in our court! Appreciating this simple concept may turn out to be one of the most empowering and liberating health pearls of all that you gain here.

Continuing on with the engine metaphor — fueling our body, and by extension our metabolism, with the best possible fuel, could be equivalent to upgrading our gasoline powered vehicle for a newer, more versatile model, that runs much more efficiently, and may be more flexible, being able to run on different fuels. Like a hybrid vehicle, for example, one that allows the vehicle to either use gasoline (petroleum-based fuel) or electricity to generate its energy and can switch between sources effortlessly.

An eight-cylinder hybrid SUV runs much more efficiently than an older, smaller, and non-hybrid vehicle. (Trust me, with my family of eight, we've had both.) It also gets much better gas mileage than previous, much smaller minivans, and does so through a much more efficient and flexible engine! It does not have a *faster* engine per se, but the fact that it goes much farther on the same tank of gas is marvelous! This is exactly what we want our bodies to be able to do: to get more out of the fuel we put in it, and be able to switch seamlessly between fuels, so that our metabolism is both flexible and efficient.

You may ask, what fuels are best for our metabolism? Great question! Sadly, much of the teaching and information on this topic of metabolism and its ideal fuel has been either lacking or inaccurate for decades. During medical school, I was taught that we must have significant amounts of sugar and carbohydrates in our diet, primarily because our brains need glucose to survive. Could this be the reason carbohydrates tend to make up the largest percentage of foods consumed worldwide?

The notion that we need glucose in order for our brains to survive, however, is only a half-truth. Our brains and our body can also use alternative fuels such as ketones, and may even actually prefer them over glucose. Ketones are produced by the liver from fats, as an alternate fuel source when the body is low on sugar or glucose stores. Many studies have shown that the brain performs better on ketones.[42] Remember the previous section on fasting and how our brain tends to be more focused and sharp? Research on disease prevention and symptom improvement using a ketogenic diet (low carb diet) has also shown utility in many chronic diseases, including epilepsy, ADHD, Alzheimer's disease, migraines, and even cancer.[43, 44, 45]

In addition to using alternative fuel sources, the necessary minimum requirement for glucose in our bloodstream can be obtained from the body's innate ability to manufacture glucose on its own in the liver, through a process called gluconeogenesis (making new glucose). This process can and does occur to help our body maintain sufficient glucose in the blood, without any additional dietary carbohydrates or sugar — a concept underappreciated within the medical field, as well as the health and fitness space.

Gluconeogenesis is what allows us the ability to withstand an overnight fast (not eating while we sleep), or a sustained multiple-day fast, as long as we are appropriately hydrated.

In other words, the only potential non-essential macronutrient in the diet is carbohydrates.

Now, I am not suggesting we completely avoid carbohydrates. I am simply saying that, technically, we can live without them, though admittedly I don't believe we should. There are many real food-based carbohydrates that come in the form of natural vegetables and fruits which can be very beneficial for our health, and add significant variety and joy. I personally look forward to the variety of bright and colorful vegetables and fruits, both fresh and fermented, that regularly make up an important and tasty part of my well crafted meal plate.

Now, please do not take this physiological truth of the non-necessity of carbohydrates at mere face value, nor make subsequent changes to your diet without first discussing your decision with your healthcare provider, especially if you are on medication(s). This is especially important to consider if you are diabetic or on blood sugar lowering medication.

With this condition, you will soon learn, if you drop your carbohydrate intake significantly, this may cause serious effects on your blood sugar and insulin levels, possibly leading to hypoglycemia (low blood sugar), if these medications are not properly adjusted under medical supervision.

So, if we are not consuming significant amounts of glucose or carbohydrates in our diet, what, then, *is* fueling us?

If it is not the carbs, then what? Well, it would be the two other macronutrients, fats and proteins, that would provide the fuel in this case. Interestingly, studies have collected data regarding which fuel source is optimal for our body, and in most cases, it's actually not glucose *or* carbohydrates. Fat, in the form of fatty acids, is the preferred fuel for the heart, and typically accounts for up to 70% of the energy, produced in the form of ATP (adenosine triphosphate) by the heart, while the remaining 30% is from glucose, protein, and ketones.[42] It may be a surprise that fats are preferred by the heart, and are more energy dense, which means more energy is provided per gram than glucose and protein.

Fats also burn cleaner. This means they produce less reactive oxygen species (ROS) or free radicals which are unstable atoms made during normal metabolism, and therefore produce less inflammation (more on this later in the macronutrient chapters). Ketones, a breakdown product of fats, which have been shown to be present during intermittent and prolonged fasting, and in aerobic exercise, can improve blood flow to the heart (myocardial perfusion), and are currently being tested as a treatment for heart failure, with promising results.[45]

There was also an interesting experiment done in the mid-1990s on the mammalian rat heart, which demonstrated that the heart beat 30% stronger and more efficiently (it had a higher cardiac output) when fats were used as fuel, as opposed to glucose![46] Many other studies have been performed demonstrating an increased understanding of the importance of fats and ketones, with respect to heart function and heart health. At the same time, more continue to look into the optimal fuel mix, as well as beneficial effects in the treatment of neurodegenerative conditions like Alzheimer's, Parkinson's, many cancers, and other conditions such as heart failure.

In addition to the superior fuel quality of fats and ketones over glucose, ketones in many cases have also been shown to decrease the oxidative stress of metabolism, leading to less inflammation and improvements in many health conditions. This is because they work as an anti-inflammatory and antioxidant protective barrier.[43, 44]

By now, you will have more reasons to consider decreasing your carbohydrate intake, and try increasing your healthy fats intake instead. In addition to behavioral modifications such as intermittent fasting, your metabolism will be on its way to becoming a re-energized machine, helping you reach your overall health goals.

But how do we determine our metabolic health? Is the one we have now in excellent condition, or is it in need of a tune-up? How can we get our metabolism tuned up and "purring," while switching effortlessly between fuel sources so that it runs in tip-top shape and is ready to crush life?

Read on, and this will soon be revealed.

Are You Metabolically Flexible or Not?

What You Need to Know:

- Getting your metabolism to function in a healthier way by fixing your cellular engines (mitochondria) to be versatile is the goal of metabolic flexibility
- Metabolic flexibility gives you more energy, burns fat, and decreases inflammation

---

So, how can you tell? Without getting too deep into the weeds, a simple test to check your metabolic flexibility is to spontaneously fast between 12–24 hours and do so without significant difficulty, while maintaining a good level of energy. If you pass, you are off to a great start. If you are able to skip two or three meals without feeling "hangry," and still be energetic enough to carry out your daily activities, then you likely have some degree of metabolic flexibility. If you are unable to do this, however, or experience significant cravings, then definitely read on!

It is not simply about exercising more to speed up your metabolism. Now, exercise is great, though better yet, if you incorporate strength or resistance training into your workout, you will then increase your muscle mass, which will correspondingly increase the number and functioning of your mitochondria, which is key to metabolism. More muscle equals more mitochondria which in turn equals more energy! Additionally, metabolic flexibility is really about getting your metabolism to function in a healthier way, by fixing your mitochondria (cellular engines) to run more efficiently.

Metabolic flexibility is your body's ability to respond or adapt to conditional changes in both metabolic demand and fuel types. Our metabolism needs to be able to adapt seamlessly to times of eating, fasting, and exercise. This concept explains what occurs when this flexibility ceases to work at peak efficiency, as the body then gravitates toward obesity and insulin resistance, for instance.

Here the processes which determine fuel selection between glucose and fats are interrupted, making it difficult to alternate between fuel sources.[30] Often the metabolism of an obese person or one experiencing insulin resistance largely runs on glucose, and not so much on fat, making it very difficult to lose that stored fat (extra weight). We may call this non-preferred state metabolic *in*flexibility.

Obviously, these conditions of inflexibility are not ideal. Having a flexible metabolism, and thus flexible mitochondria which can alternate between fuel sources, is a much healthier and cleaner way to function. This not only leads to better and longer-lasting energy production, but less damaging waste product formation — commonly in the form of damaging free radicals — which promote inflammation and cellular damage in the mitochondria. Metabolic flexibility not only gives you more energy and burns fat, but also leads to less inflammation. This is a true win-win!

Let's talk more for a moment about the little guys called mitochondria. Why should we care about these microscopic entities, anyway? Because they are the *most important* players in our metabolism. Nearly all the energy we have ever made, from all the calories we have ever consumed, from all the food we have ever eaten throughout our entire lives, has been made primarily inside our mitochondria. They are truly our body's power plants and energy sources. To have no mitochondria would equal death! So, do you think we should consider improving the health, efficiency, and flexibility of our mitochondria? Absolutely!

Mitochondria are quite literally the "powerhouses or power plants" of all the cells in our bodies. They are small organelles (small organs) inside our cells that play a key role in our metabolic health, as well as our complete health and wellness. Optimizing our mitochondrial health not only gives us more energy, but also helps us avoid many chronic diseases.[47]

These cellular engines inside virtually every cell in our body produce the energy required for all the metabolic processes that keep us alive, including converting the food we eat, and the air we breathe, into energy. They are single-handedly the most important energy factory in our body, and are the most important to our metabolism. Each and every cell in our body needs energy to survive, and most of that energy is produced inside of these mitochondria.

112

Our mitochondrial health is not only directly connected to the health of our *metabolism*, but is also key to our *overall* health. If things go awry in our mitochondria (largely due to poor food choices, or other harmful exposures and behavioral practices), we will be prone to becoming overweight, struggling with obesity, as well as a myriad of chronic diseases — insulin and leptin resistance, full-blown diabetes, heart disease, and cancer — to name a few.

The way we care for our mitochondria is the most important aspect of metabolic health. After all, they are the power plants of our cells, and are the primary location for energy production in the body. Without energy, we are dead.

One simple, yet critical, way we care for them is by the food choices we make every day. Remember food can be the best fuel and medicine or a slow poison. And these mitochondria respond directly and obligatorily to the foods we eat. Feeding them fuel that burns the cleanest and is best for ideal energy production, while producing less damaging waste, is one way to care for our mitochondria. Natural healthy fats, instead of processed carbohydrates and seed oils, are a better choice for metabolic health.[48]

These natural, unprocessed fats can be found in whole foods such as avocados, coconuts, and olives, especially extra virgin olive oil, as well as from well-sourced, pesticide, hormone, antibiotic, and additive-*free* animal fat and animal products (butter, ghee, tallow, suet, etc.). On the contrary, highly processed foods, grains, sugars, and seed oils (vegetable oils such as canola, corn, cottonseed, safflower, sunflower, soybean, grapeseed and rice-bran oils) "burn dirty" in these cellular engines, and generate a lot of waste or damaging end products — free radicals and reactive oxygen species — which ultimately produce significant and harmful inflammation which damages mitochondria and therefore metabolism. Having a high-functioning, versatile, and clean burning metabolism *is* possible, and starts with what lies at the end of our fork!

Given we are talking about metabolic flexibility, let's pause for a moment to address metabolic syndrome, one of the leading contributors to coronary heart disease. Think of it as a physical demonstration of a wrecked metabolism, or a poorly functioning one. According to the Mayo Clinic, it is defined as a cluster of conditions that often occur together, which increase your risk of heart disease, stroke, and type 2 diabetes.[0] These conditions include elevated blood pressure or hypertension, elevated blood sugar (diabetes, pre-diabetes, or insulin resistance), excess body fat around the waist (the so-called visceral fat), and elevated levels of cholesterol and triglycerides.

Having just one of these conditions does not necessarily mean you have full-blown metabolic syndrome, but it may indicate a greater risk of developing it, as well as other serious health conditions. Metabolic syndrome is becoming increasingly common. One-third of U.S. adults have it, and almost 90% of all adults have at least one feature of it.[3] Fortunately, it is largely preventable and modifiable, and you can change this!

It is almost entirely under your control. With aggressive lifestyle changes (described throughout this book), it can be delayed, and even entirely prevented.[49]

Similarly common is the prevalence of insulin resistance, which according to Dr. Benjamin Bikman may occur in up to eighty-eight percent of the U.S. population.[50] Insulin resistance is one of the first signs of a damaged and inflexible metabolism. It is a leading proponent of obesity, and one of the most common diseases today.

You may ask, "What is insulin resistance, anyway?" Let me explain.

Insulin Resistance

What You Need to Know:

- Insulin controls whether carbs or fats will be used as energy or stored as fat
- An inability of one's cells to properly process sugars is the root of many health conditions
- Insulin resistance can be reversed through diet and lifestyle changes
- Lower insulin levels ensure normal fat burning, decreased cravings, and more energy

Normally, your digestive system breaks down the carbohydrates you eat into sugar or glucose. The hormone insulin, produced by your pancreas, then helps ensure the sugar enters your cells to be used as fuel or stored as fat. In people with insulin resistance, cells do not respond normally to insulin, and glucose does not enter the cells as easily. As a result, your blood sugar (glucose) levels rise, even as your body churns out more and more insulin to try to lower your blood sugar.

Insulin is a master hormone, and if you have a resistance to it, you may also have other hormonal problems. Insulin resistance by itself is connected to numerous other hormonal imbalances. These may include polycystic ovary syndrome

(PCOS), premature menopause, low testosterone (low T), thyroid problems, and adrenal issues, which can all have their roots in insulin resistance. It is a common problem worldwide.

I prefer to put a positive spin on insulin resistance.

> *By taking preventative measures, we can improve and even potentially cure many of the hormonal imbalances associated with insulin resistance.*

With it being the root of many health conditions we as humanity face, treating it could potentially reverse our suffering! And I have seen exactly this in my practice.

One great example is the case of one of my thirty-year-old female patients with PCOS and infertility. When we focused on treating her insulin resistance through diet and lifestyle modification, her PCOS went away and she was able to get pregnant. Miraculous, maybe, but it exemplifies the power of this master hormone, insulin, and the benefits of optimizing its effects on overall health.

You may ask, "If insulin resistance is so common, how do I know if I have it?" Unfortunately, despite its common presence in most of the population — up to 88% of us, as alluded to previously — from my experience, most physicians overlook this prevalence. And what happens if we don't look for something? We can't find it! This may be the fate faced by *many* patients, whose physicians are not aware of the epidemic that is insulin resistance.

In medical school, there was not much, if any, focus on insulin and insulin resistance, beyond the simple relationship of insulin to blood sugar. That is to say that when blood sugar rises, the prescribed treatment is always to get more insulin, in an attempt to lower the blood sugar. What was tested for then, and commonly now, was not insulin, but the level of blood sugar or glucose. This test misses the diagnosis of most cases of insulin resistance until the onset of quite advanced, nearly full-blown diabetes.

My guess is if you ask your doctor to check your insulin level (as I asked my doctor last year), you may experience the same "eye roll" I got from my personal physician, and be told that this is not a standard test. Instead, he or she may just check your blood sugar. Yet simply checking blood sugar as a screening test for insulin resistance will miss most cases of this disease. Therefore, insist on checking a *fasting* insulin level!

Once you have your fasting insulin and blood sugar levels (ideally you would get them drawn at the same time, after an eight-hour overnight fast), you can then do a simple calculation, called the Homeostatic Model Assessment for Insulin Resistance (HOMA-IR). This will allow you to get an idea if you are insulin resistant or not. This can be achieved by using an online medical calculator or by simply computing it yourself with the following equation:

[Glucose in (mg/dL) x Insulin (microUnits/mL)] / 405 (here in the U.S.)

or

[Glucose in mmol/L x Insulin in microUnits/ml] / 22.5 (for the majority of other countries)

Although there is no absolute consensus on the cutoff score, having a HOMA-IR less than one is ideal. Greater than 1.5 is early insulin resistance (IR), and greater than 3 is considered significant insulin resistance, or borderline type 2 diabetes.[50]

The ability to measure insulin was discovered more than fifty years ago in the late 1950s. And despite the availability of the insulin blood test, it is rarely used today, even though it could help to diagnose diabetes up to twenty years earlier than by using the common method of an elevated glucose level for diagnosis.[51]

The diagnosis of both type 1 and type 2 diabetes has been focused largely on the presence of elevated blood sugar or glucose in a simple blood test. And the ultimate treatment of these two very different diseases eventually ends with insulin administration.

Type 1 diabetes, or what was traditionally referred to as juvenile-onset diabetes, is typically caused by too little insulin due to dysfunctional beta cells in the pancreas, which are responsible for producing insulin. This can be caused by various mechanisms of inflammation or injury to the pancreas, all of which ultimately have the same result: the pancreas is unable to produce sufficient insulin to respond to blood glucose, and therefore blood sugar (glucose) rises on the account of little or no insulin.

Type 2 diabetes, in sharp contrast to type 1, is typically demonstrated by very elevated insulin levels. Though insulin levels can be many times the normal limit, the blood sugar still rises, because insulin resistance prevents the insulin from properly working.

Why, then, are these two very different types of diabetes treated so similarly in mainstream medicine, if they are nearly opposite in their etiology? This is a great question, because there *is* a better way!

Treating two completely different diseases the same way, with insulin, is fraught with problems. And as health care professionals, we can do better. Giving insulin to someone with type 2 diabetes, who already has elevated insulin levels in their blood, is not the best option, and in my experience can exacerbate the insulin resistance and weight gain they are attempting to treat.

By also affecting other hormones: glucagon; human growth hormone (HGH); adrenalin; estrogen; testosterone; thyroid hormone, and others, insulin is considered a master hormone. Largely controlling our metabolism as it does, it is therefore paramount for our insulin to remain at normal levels, in order to thus have a properly functioning metabolism (a metabolism that's not broken) — with no significant insulin resistance.

In relation to our metabolism, insulin almost single-handedly determines whether fats or glucose get released into the bloodstream to be used as fuel, or whether it gets stored in the cells as fat. Simply stated, when insulin levels are up, the body enters an anabolic or fat storage mode, and when insulin levels remain low, fat comes out of storage, and can be used as fuel.

Many studies link elevated insulin levels, or hyperinsulinemia, to not only this fat-building mode, but also to carbohydrate craving, hyperphagia (increased appetite or frequent eating), decreased fat burning, and decreased physical energy.53 Generally speaking, having low insulin levels allows for just the opposite: decreased cravings and more satiety, fat burning rather than fat storing, and increased physical energy. It is therefore important to maintain a lower level of insulin, in order to burn that stubborn body fat and experience wonderful effects of decreased cravings, less hunger, and more energy.

Conversely, when insulin is high, the body uses glucose and fatty acids to build, fatten, and grow new fat cells, rather than burn them for energy — this, in turn, makes us fatter. As discussed, elevated insulin levels have been linked to obesity.[53] What is also very interesting is that this process of storing glucose as fat is not as easily reversed as we may like it to be.

What do I mean by this? Well, have you ever experienced difficulty losing body fat, despite working hard with exercise and your diet, and you just can't get those stubborn few pounds or inches around the midsection to melt away? If so, you are not alone, and there is a physiologic reason for this. It is not misfortune or merely the fact that you are getting older. When that fat was created, largely from sugar or carbohydrates, it was a simple and straightforward process:

Insulin controls whether carbohydrates and fat will be used for energy or stored as fat!

It's that simple! Insulin's main role is to remove glucose from the bloodstream and put it into fat cells for storage. Turning the glucose into fat for storage tends to be a much simpler process than taking that same stored energy as fat out of the adipose cells, and breaking it down into usable energy, which involves low insulin levels, among other things.

Many of us consume carbohydrates throughout the day (think of those snacks in between meals), which raises our blood sugar and corresponding insulin levels. It then becomes nearly impossible to access and use that stored fat for energy, because of the elevated insulin shifting the balance towards fat storage mode. And as long as insulin levels are high, it is nearly impossible to burn fat — you are not likely to shed those extra pounds. At the end of the day, those carb-filled snacks we love so much sabotage our weight loss goals, keeping us insulin resistant.

And which outcome do you want?

The good news is: this is under your control! In due course, we will further discuss the important concept of macronutrients: carbohydrates, proteins, and fats. We will then specifically discuss what can be done to keep our insulin levels low, so that we can actually burn that stubborn body fat, and lose those inches, while simultaneously providing our bodies with the most efficient and long-lasting energy source to fuel us all day long!

But first, let us take a trip into the crazy life of carbohydrates. Why do we crave them? And do we *really* need to include them in a diet that enables overall health?

The Crazy Topic of Carbohydrates

What You Need to Know:

- Digested carbohydrates are broken down into glucose or sugar
- Consuming natural carbs like veggies, fruit, and berries can be a great addition to any diet
- Avoid ready-to-eat processed foods — they contain highly processed, refined grains and sugars (carbohydrates), and often unhealthy seed oils
- Fiber containing "slow" carbs have healthier benefits than blood sugar elevating "fast" carbs

I'll start our macronutrient discussion with none other than carbohydrates. Why? Because they are not only a lot of fun to discuss, but tend to be the least well understood in the health space. They are also the most common macronutrient consumed by most cultures worldwide.

Carbs are not the devil.

Instead, *carbs are carbs,* and are not inherently good or bad. To say there is a lot of misinformation circulating about carbohydrates is an understatement. They continue to be recommended by the USDA as the primary nutrient of consumption (45–65% of total daily Calories)[54], though personally I disagree with this recommendation.

When digested, carbohydrates, regardless of the source, are essentially broken down into glucose or sugar, and if insulin remains elevated, then most commonly are stored as fat. When we talk about blood sugar, we mean glucose, which is the most basic carbohydrate.

Let's review some basic carbohydrate biochemistry. Now, I urge you not to tune out, go to sleep, or skip this. I promise to keep it simple, and it will be *worth it.*

Carbohydrates simply contain three basic elements: Carbon, Hydrogen, and Oxygen. All three are essentially broken down into simpler sugars, and ultimately glucose. Carbohydrates play a very important role in the human body. They act as an energy source, help control blood glucose and insulin metabolism, participate in cholesterol and triglyceride metabolism, and play a key part in metabolic health. However, only about 4% of the energy produced from carbohydrates can be stored as glucose (glycogen), and up to 96% of the energy is stored as fat![55]

Did you know that your body can actually live off a diet largely devoid of carbohydrates? Yes, you heard that right. You do not have to consume many, if any, carbs to survive. Your body can make the limited glucose that it needs in the liver in a process called gluconeogenesis, and your brain will have sufficient glucose via this naturally produced mechanism!

This is not to say that you should not have carbs at all. Personally, I find that consuming the right kinds, natural ones like vegetables, fruit and berries, can be a beautiful and wonderful part of any diet. But no, you do not *actually* need any added carbs in your diet for survival. Crazy, huh? I know this may not be well publicized in nutrition or medical science spaces, but it is true.

I do not make the point that we don't need dietary carbohydrates for survival to understate their role in our diet.

> *There are a lot of good carbs out there in the form of fresh, whole, real food that comes with added vitamins, minerals, fiber, and antioxidants: fresh fruit, nuts, and vegetables, for example.*

So why are carbs getting a bad reputation these days? Well, we now know that they ultimately become sugar in our bodies, causing blood glucose and insulin to rise. This simple fact is true of all carbohydrates. Sugar is sugar, yes? So carbohydrates are sugar then, right? Well, yes and no.

NOT ALL carbohydrates are created equal. Carbohydrates are found in just about every food group: fruits and vegetables, grains and dairy, and are even found in protein-rich legumes and nuts. Even so, some are healthier than others.

The worst offenders in the category of carbohydrates may in fact be the highly processed and refined ones that are found in most ready-to-eat foods we buy at the supermarket (those that come in a **Box**, **Bag**, or with a **Barcode** – 'the three B's'). These highly refined and processed carbohydrates are not great. One reason is due to the highly processed and refined nature of these types, and how this affects digestion. The second is that most of these processed foods contain not-so-awesome chemical ingredients like the seed oils.

Seed oils are those highly processed vegetable oils that, although technically plant-based, tend to be high in inflammatory polyunsaturated fatty acids (PUFAs) such as canola, corn, cottonseed, soy, safflower, rice-bran, grapeseed, and sunflower oil. These seed oils are terrible for us and our metabolism, because of the tremendous inflammation they cause, among various other things. We will delve more into this when we turn to the topic of fats.

It is better to eat carbohydrates from real, whole, natural, organic, and non-GMO foods. It is also better, still, to eat more of what I refer to as the "slow" carbs than the "fast."

Say what?

What is a "fast" and a "slow" carb?

"Slow" carbs can be defined as those found in natural foods, which also tend to come with fiber, like those in fresh whole fruits and vegetables, as well as naturally unrefined whole grains, nuts, and seeds. Due to their additional fiber content, they tend to take longer to digest, therefore causing a "slower" rise in blood sugar. These fiber-containing "slow" carbs tend to prevent us from feeling so hungry shortly after eating them — in complete contrast to the processed and refined carbohydrates which I refer to as the "fast" carbs.

These are often found in highly processed foods: white and wheat bread, pasta, and baked goods (chips, cookies, crackers, cakes, and other goodies), most breakfast cereals, granola, sugary drinks like soda and juices, and other sweet treats. They are not only typically devoid of natural fiber and many other healthy nutrients, but they also cause a rapid rise in blood sugar and a concomitant rise in insulin.

These types of "fast" carbs leave you feeling hungry, tired, and craving more shortly after eating them. This is because of the rapid rise and then fall in glucose which can lead to a symptomatic hypoglycemia as the blood sugar drops rapidly after its peak causing low energy, the "hangry" feeling and cravings for more carbs. Remember, these are the carbs that spike our glucose and insulin levels, causing our bodies to store the glucose as fat and develop insulin resistance, which is something we don't want.

The Glycemic Index (GI) is a helpful tool that also aids in characterizing whether a carbohydrate will likely be a "fast" or "slow" carb. It is a relative ranking of carbohydrates in foods, according to how they typically affect blood glucose levels. Using the Glycemic Index can help to wisely choose the carbohydrates we consume. It is usually broken down into three categories or levels: Low is described as a GI of 55 or below which would tend to be a "slow" carb, Moderate is 56 to 69, and High is 70 and above which would fall into the "fast" carb category.

Carbohydrates with a lower GI value tend to be more slowly digested, absorbed, and metabolized, and will cause a lower and slower rise in blood glucose. This would typically be the natural whole fruits, vegetables, and legumes which we have referred to as the "slow" carbs.

Let me give you a few examples:

Some natural carbohydrates with a lower GI (0-55) are:

A raw apple (36); raw grapefruit (25); raw cherries (20); raw pear, orange, peach, and strawberries (all in the 40-43 range); carrots (39); vegetable soup (49); chickpeas (28); kidney beans (24), and lentils (32).*

Now compare this to more processed foods, such as:

Standard whole wheat or white bread (75+); white rice (73); brown rice (68); breakfast cereal such as cornflakes (81), and instant oats (79) versus plain rolled oats (55).*

The bottom line is one should try to consume sugar or carbohydrates naturally from fresh vegetables, fruits, and legumes as much as possible, while avoiding the processed ones.

Notice that I did not add any fruit juices to the list of 'slow carbs'? That is because most juices — natural, organic, or not — tend to have much less fiber than if you eat the whole fruit. Juices tend to cause your blood sugar, and later insulin, to spike much higher than if you were to eat the same fruit in its whole form. **Therefore, I usually recommend *eating* your fruit, and *not drinking* it.**

You may ask why bread has a much higher GI than that of vegetables and fruit, when its ingredients seem fairly simple. Well, the wheat flour is so finely ground and processed that it gives the digestive enzymes a much greater surface area with which to interact and metabolize the bread. A general lack of high-quality nutrients in most processed bread means they often do not require any significant digestive processing, which would slow things down, and instead rapidly spike the blood sugar. Two examples of healthier bread would be natural sprouted bread (GI from 36-40) or freshly made sourdough bread from an organic starter (GI around 50). Beyond this, most breads available in the U.S. come from GMO hybridized dwarf wheat which is typically pesticide laden and has a much higher percentage of gluten and related allergenic compounds than do the buckwheat or other less hybridized wheats used in other European countries, for example. For this reason, I rarely eat breads in the U.S. unless they are sprouted, gluten free, and devoid of GMO ingredients. However, I can tolerate much better the natural sourdoughs and better grain, less processed, breads in the Mediterranean when I have traveled there.

You may also wonder if there are any optimization habits that can be applied if you simply *must* have a certain carbohydrate you enjoy. Well, there are a few ways to delay the spike of glucose and resulting insulin after eating carbohydrates. When you add other items to your meal, such as fat or protein, this will generally prolong the digestive process. This causes a slower spike of glucose and insulin, which overall may lower the Glycemic Index of your meal. In other words, don't eat your carbs *naked* or *alone*. Instead, eat them with healthy natural fats and proteins. Delaying the carbs to the end of the meal also leads to a lower and less steep spike in blood sugar and corresponding insulin as well; in this way starting your meal with protein or healthy fats and leaving carbohydrates until *later* in the meal is quite helpful too.

Additionally, adding acidic foods such as lemon juice, apple cider vinegar, pickles, or fermenting carbohydrates (sourdough bread made from a starter) can also lower the GI of your meal and concomitant blood sugar and insulin spike. Other great fermented carbohydrates to consider adding to your menu are kimchi, sauerkraut, kefir, tempeh, natto, miso, kombucha, and yogurt. Not only will they decrease the spike of glucose and insulin, but they are packed with natural probiotics and more readily bioavailable nutrients.

Now let's look at how well and for how long carbohydrates can fuel us. To understand this better, knowing a few of the different amounts of calories burned during certain activities can be helpful. For example, typical numbers for Calories burned at rest are 1–2 Calories per minute while seated, and a bit more while standing, and 3–4 Calories per minute doing light work such as errands in an office.

Say you had a bagel, scone, or croissant for breakfast (primarily composed of processed carbohydrates), which would be broken down into sugar. This could power you for 2–2 1/2 hours maximum, if your energy expenditure consisted of doing light office work! Now you know why you feel hungry so quickly, even before lunch!

I have realized that if I eat a bagel, scone, or croissant (often the food available at a hospital cafeteria or early morning hospital meeting) they leave me feeling hungry an hour or two later. However, if I have an egg (or three!) and a slice of minimally processed sprouted bread, or natural sourdough from a starter, toasted with avocado on top, I'm good until lunch. (This is due to "dressing" my carbs with protein and healthy fats — coming from the eggs and avocado — rather than eating the toast or bagel "naked," or alone.)

So, this is where things start making sense. If we have a diet of mostly carbohydrates, we will feel hungry all the time, and gain weight (as when insulin is up, and our glycogen stores have been met, which happens very readily, then the glucose or carbs will get stored as fat). You may have heard the phrase, "it's not the fat that makes you fat, it's the carbs or sugar that make you fat!" This is correct, and now you know why!

On the other hand, if you primarily eat fat or protein without many carbs, you won't have to succumb to the significant glucose and corresponding insulin spike, that is ultimately making you fat! Fat or protein is much more satiating, and not only leaves you feeling full for a much longer period of time, but provides you with longer-lasting, cleaner energy!

Remember that fat is your body's most concentrated energy source, providing more than double the energy as carbohydrates or protein (fat contains approximately nine Calories per gram, versus four Calories per gram from carbohydrates or glucose). When using fat primarily for fuel, blood carries about sixty Calories at a time while at rest, and can increase ten-fold with exercise!

That's significantly more energy available than if you are primarily using carbohydrates for fuel — about quadruple the energy available at rest, and then forty times more during exercise! This is the energy secret: burning fat can melt those stubborn pounds and inches, while primarily burning carbohydrates will likely not. We will get into this in much greater detail very soon.

For now, I will leave you with a quick pearl on how to avoid the trap of carbohydrate or sugar addiction, which often comes in the form of "snacking." Remember that carbs simply do not satiate us, and can only supply us with brief non-sustained energy, leaving us starved for energy from a metabolic standpoint, and causing us to crave more of them. This carb craving and carb dependence is a sign of a broken or metabolically inflexible metabolism.

The good news is that your metabolism can quickly recover from this dependency on carbohydrates for fuel, by taking simple actions. To begin, stop unhealthy snacking! It will pay huge dividends to your overall health. Eating real whole food, not processed and refined carbohydrates, and adding more satiating proteins and healthy fats to your diet, will also jumpstart this process. Incorporating some specific timing rituals to eating, like intermittent fasting or time-restricted feeding, will also lend a huge boost to fixing your metabolism, taking you from a *carbohydrate-fueled* to *flexible* metabolism.

Fats DO NOT Make You Fat

What You Need to Know:

- Natural fats from plant and animal sources have huge benefits
- Learning the difference between "good" and "bad" fat is simply understanding that good is natural and bad is processed

---

This can be a very controversial and quite confusing topic within the diet and nutritional spaces. Research data and subsequent recommendations regarding fats and cholesterol have completely changed several times in my lifetime. I grew up in the middle of the 1970s and 80s when the nutritional dogma that fat, especially saturated fat and cholesterol (from natural things like butter and eggs), was believed to cause heart disease.

At the same time, it was believed that the plant-derived artificial fats from vegetable and seed oils (corn, canola, cottonseed, soy, safflower, sunflower, grapeseed, ricebran, and others), in addition to margarine and fake fats (hydrogenated oils), were better for you. Nothing could be further from the truth!

Today, the health community accepts the benefits natural fats from plant and animal sources have to offer. Pressed avocado, coconut, and extra virgin olive oils, as well as butter from grass-fed cows, ghee, lard and tallow, and well-sourced eggs, have huge benefits.

The dangers of artificial butters and oils, on the other hand, though derived from plants, lie in their polyunsaturated fatty acids (PUFAs), and hydrogenated oils: margarine, vegetable shortenings, plant-based spreads, and seed oils. Unaware of their detrimental effects to our metabolism, many people continue to consume these plant-based spreads and oils at alarmingly high rates. And all the more disturbingly, they are in the overwhelming majority of processed foods, sauces, and dressings!

The nutritional teachings in the 60s, 70s, and 80s to this day have my mother believing eggs and butter are bad for you. She nearly has a heart attack when I tell her I regularly eat four eggs a day, despite me saying that they are a great source of natural protein and healthy cholesterol, which is not only essential but amazing for our brain and overall health! My mom still believes highly processed, plant-based fake butter spreads and oils (especially if they are organic) must be better for us.

In this chapter, we will take a deep dive into all things FAT and CHOLESTEROL. Not only to dispel these decades-old myths, but also to empower you to healthily eat fat and cholesterol — which are among the best possible fuels for our metabolism!

Let's start with that which my mother fears most — cholesterol! Believe it or not, cholesterol is essential for our optimal brain and total body health. It is not to be feared. We actually *need* cholesterol, and *cannot live* without it. It is that important! If we don't incorporate it into our diet, our body will move heaven and earth to produce it. Cholesterol is that vital.

So why have we demonized it?

Fat is not the enemy!
Fat does not necessarily make you fat!
Fat or cholesterol themselves are not the problems!

In my evaluation of the available evidence, the low fat craze and stigma against saturated fat was created not by good scientific evidence, but by a highly charged opinion agenda and propaganda. The actual data used to create this dogma was never supported by high-quality evidence, like that of randomized controlled trials (RCT). Any true scientific basis or support for the USDA Food Guidelines or health recommendations, that specifically recommend cutting fat in the diet (especially natural saturated fat), does not exist.[57, 58] I repeat, there is no good prospective scientific data to support the USDA recommendations to cut fat; especially natural saturated fat. None.

Despite having no solid scientific evidence to support these dietary guidelines (to cut fat and saturated fat to less than 30% and 10% of the total diet, respectively), this recommendation by the USDA has often created an unwarranted fear of fat and cholesterol. This has caused many people to substitute healthy fat options with processed carbohydrates and poor quality, plant-based vegetable and seed oils (high in PUFA-rich omega-6 fatty acids) — likely the root of our obesity epidemic and skyrocketing heart disease statistics.

The simple reality is that when you have only three major macronutrients — fat, carbohydrate, and protein — and then significantly reduce the quantity of one of them in the diet, you tend to increase the amount of one or two of the remaining. When fat is being cut, this usually corresponds with eating more carbohydrates. Typically, the least healthy carbohydrates tend to be those readily available, that come in a package with a label. We talked in the previous chapter about how these carbohydrates are not necessarily good for us.

Remember, in the U.S. alone, more than 70% of the population is overweight, and more than 40% can be classified as obese![13] These numbers have significantly increased over the last fifty years, since the USDA published its original recommendations to lower fat intake. And how is this low-fat dietary recommendation working out? Not very well.

I find it curious that in fifty years of U.S. government involvement with food guidelines, recommending significantly cutting fat (specifically saturated fat), the United States' obesity rates rose to new heights, making the U.S. one of the fattest countries on the planet. Coincidence? Perhaps. But agenda, politics, and poor science seem to have also combined together in this perfect storm of poor dietary choices.

The latest iteration of the USDA dietary guidelines for 2020–2025 still contains these same low-fat dietary recommendations which have failed miserably, and have no doubt since the recommendations began, contributed to the worst obesity epidemic in the history of the U.S.[59]

De Souza et al. reported in 2015, in a large meta-analysis, that there was no association between saturated fats and increased all-cause mortality, Cardiovascular Disease (CVD), Coronary Heart Disease (CHD), ischemic stroke, or type 2 diabetes.[60] In other words, saturated fat was not to blame for increasing rates of these ailments.

This is in complete contradiction to Ancel Keys' unsubstantiated work from the 1950s-1970s on the premise that saturated fats cause heart disease, subsequent USDA nutrition guidelines, and the popular fat and cholesterol dogma of the last half-century. Several other meta-analyses also support this conclusion: saturated fat is not to blame for the increase in cardiovascular disease (CVD), coronary heart disease (CHD), stroke, or diabetes.[61, 62]

To summarize, Ancel Keys not only cherry-picked his data, but also ignored the data that did not support his theory.[63] The data he did choose to use he misinterpreted, and made deceptive causation conclusions when it was not possible to do so with the epidemiological data he collected. As a result, his efforts may be one of the primary reasons we, as a Western society, have gotten ourselves into this low-fat paradigm that still perpetuates today.

Besides Ancel Keys severely misleading us with his cherry-picked data, potentially causing us to fear fats, the greatest error was perhaps that in the interim fifty years the PUFAs like seed oils (which are highly inflammatory and dangerous to health) were promoted, while the healthier and more natural fats: coconut, avocado, butter, ghee, tallow, and suet were demonized.

When you dig deep into this history, it may or may not be a surprise to you that the USDA and other large organizations such as the American Heart Association (AHA) have taken considerable funding from the big food manufacturers (think Proctor and Gamble, among others) and pharmaceutical companies (think cholesterol-lowering drug manufacturers) which both benefit from this low-fat paradigm.

In fact, many of the key studies on LDL (low-density lipoproteins) and cholesterol were sponsored by pharmaceutical companies, whose main goal may have been to find a venue to promote and recommend cholesterol-lowering medications. This not only would ensure their long-term survival and profitability at that time, but for decades to come. Did they accomplish this? Unfortunately, yes. In fact, it has been estimated that over 200 million people worldwide take one class of cholesterol-lowering medications: statins.[64]

The aftermath of this propaganda and misinformation still clouds the picture of what is healthy. Catastrophic to human health, this travesty exemplifies how food manufacturers and the government have changed the course of history, for the worse.[63]

Let me conclude by reiterating that there is no reliable scientific evidence to suggest that natural saturated fat from plant or animal sources makes us fat and causes heart disease. Neither of these are true — it's that simple. The natural unprocessed fat, both plant and animal, is actually one of the best fuels for our metabolism.

Now, we shall delve deeper into the controversy of cholesterol, and why we absolutely need it.

Why We Absolutely Need Cholesterol

What You Need to Know:

- Cholesterol is essential to our diet and our overall health
- One-quarter of our body's cholesterol is found in the brain, making it an essential contributor to our brain health
- Low-density lipoproteins (LDL) are labeled as the "bad" cholesterol protein marker
- High-density lipoproteins (HDL) are labeled as the "good" cholesterol protein marker
- More important than these lipoprotein markers is perhaps the Triglyceride to HDL ratio, and the fractionated cholesterol numbers and their particle size

---

Let's jump back to the discussion on cholesterol we began when I introduced the topic of fat. Cholesterol, like fat, is essential! It's a type of fat that we require in order to survive, we would literally die without it! Yes, believe it or not, cholesterol is actually necessary for our health, and if we are not supplied enough of it within our diet, our bodies will manufacture it anyway! It is that important!

Cholesterol is primarily made in the liver through enzymatic processes, with the rate-limiting step controlled by the enzyme HMG-CoA reductase. This enzyme may sound a little familiar to you science buffs out there, as it is the one targeted by the very common and hugely profitable class of cholesterol-lowering medication called statins.

But as we have discussed already, cholesterol in and of itself is essential to life, and not the enemy. Cholesterol is truly vital, because it is needed to form the protective phospholipid lining of all of our cells, which are the basic building blocks of our tissues and organs. It is also the chief building block of many of our hormones, including testosterone and estrogen, as well as our adrenal steroid hormones like cortisol.

Cholesterol is also essential for the production of vitamin D, one of my all-time favorite vitamins. Vitamin D is a fat-soluble, hormone-like vitamin that acts mechanistically as a steroid hormone. It goes straight to the main control center of the cell, called the nucleus, to turn on and off the genes important for maintaining bone health, immunity, and brain function, to name a few. Unfortunately, it is estimated that up to 70% of those residing in North America are deficient in vitamin D, despite its truly essential and beneficial effects. Furthermore, a study done recently during the pandemic showed that up to 82% of hospitalized patients with COVID-19 were deficient in Vitamin D.[209]

Fortunately, we are finally getting the message (in light of the recent pandemic) of the power and importance of vitamin D, as it not only increases bone and brain health, but is a significant contributor to the health of our immune system. And believe it or not, cholesterol is the basic building block from which vitamin D is made.

Cholesterol is also essential to the production of the bile acids and salts that help us digest our food — mainly the fats which help us absorb certain important nutrients like the fat-soluble vitamins of A, K, E, and of course, D. In addition, bile acids and salts are important in helping to trap and eliminate toxins from our body, which is a key factor in sustaining life and reaching optimal health.

This is especially important as there are increasing numbers of toxins in our environment, known and unknown, which can wreak havoc on our metabolism and our health. I will provide a very short list of some of the common toxins we are exposed to as humans, as a comprehensive list is beyond the scope of this book. Yet I believe a few are worth mentioning, because some of us are regularly exposed to them.

They are:

- Bisphenol A (BPA), which may be found in plastics
- Mercury, found in many fish, especially the larger ones (less so in sardines and anchovies)
- Lead and other heavy metals, which may be found in paint and polluted waters and crops cultivated therein
- Phthalates, found in many plastics
- Pesticides, such as glyphosate, found in numerous foods, especially those grown non-organically, and GMO foods
- Polychlorinated biphenyls (found in many farm-raised fish)

- Arsenic, found in soil and in some brown rice and rice syrup as well as polluted waters and some seafood
- Parabens and oxybenzone, found in many sunscreens and other cosmetic products

For more on products, their potential toxins, and overall safety concerns, please visit EWG.org, which is a great resource by the Environmental Working Group.

Our adrenal glands also need cholesterol to make our adrenal hormones like cortisol and aldosterone. The LDL (low-density lipoprotein) is also required, as it is the transport protein which carries the cholesterol to the adrenal glands, ovaries, and testes, to be able to make the necessary hormones. Therefore, LDL is absolutely necessary for life, and not exactly the enemy it is often made out to be.

Fasting, which can be so good for our health, may also increase cholesterol levels in the blood. This occurs because, when you fast, you may go into a fat-burning state. In this state, you need the LDL to perform its transport function, and bring fatty acids and cholesterol to the muscles to be used for energy. It also makes sense that an increased LDL commonly detected within a low-carb or keto diet is due to the LDL performing its carrier function, and not having anything to do with heart disease.

Though the LDL may be at the scene of a heart attack or coronary thrombosis (clogged blood vessel), it likely will not have caused the endothelial injury cascade, inflammation and associated blood clot. Instead, inflammation and oxidation due to poor diet and lifestyle factors are more likely causes of heart disease. In other words, inflammation causing the oxidized LDL to form is likely what is to blame, not the normal healthy transport LDL that is required to move the cholesterol throughout the body. I think you get the picture.

Consider this analogy. Firefighters are often found at the scene of a fire, doing their job, trying to put the fire out. Though if you take a snapshot of their presence at any given fire, and note that every time there is a fire the firefighters are also found at the scene, you could erroneously conclude, based on this snapshot in time, that they caused the fire! It sounds crazy, but this may be comparable to the LDL's relationship to heart disease.

Cholesterol is indeed very important and essential to our health, and likely not the lone culprit of heart disease or stroke. Inflammation may ultimately be to blame, as that is what oxidizes the LDL to begin with, which correlates to heart disease. This oxidized LDL caused by inflammation is what we need to be concerned with, not the LDL particle in and of itself, which simply acts as a carrier molecule. So, how do we prevent inflammation?

> *Eating an anti-inflammatory diet composed of natural, real whole foods is a good place to start.*

Highly processed and refined foods and seed oils are severely inflammatory, *not* the naturally occurring, unprocessed healthy fats and natural cholesterol.

Another super important function of cholesterol is that it is crucial to our brain health. Nearly twenty-five percent of the cholesterol in the body is actually found in the brain! In addition, elevated cholesterol levels have actually been shown to correlate with improved brain health and memory.[61] Watch out statins! The converse may also be true, that lowering cholesterol significantly (with the use, for example, of certain medications) may actually be detrimental to brain and behavioral health.

In fact, a recent study looked at the association of low LDL cholesterol levels with brain health. It was found that, especially with evidence of elevated blood pressure, having low LDL cholesterol numbers was associated with diminished brain health, specifically decreased memory and size of the gray matter in the frontal lobes (where the executive or thinking brain functions reside).

Not interested in shrinking your brain? Losing your memory? I'm with you! I strive for normal blood pressure and cholesterol levels within the normal range. And as it appears, the combination of elevated blood pressure and low cholesterol levels is not healthy for the brain. For the sake of your brain health, it is reasonable to not purposely lower your cholesterol levels through pharmaceutical means, unless there is a good indication to do so. There are natural alternatives to maintaining a healthy cholesterol level.

If you happen to be on cholesterol-lowering medications, you may want to discuss with your healthcare provider the possible side effects of this class of medications. Personally, I have seen many harmful effects of these cholesterol-lowering medications, and have dissuaded some of my personal friends and family, including my father, from taking them.

Because I believe there is another way, one that is far better and more natural. This can be accomplished by simply replacing processed carbohydrate-rich foods with healthy fats, and eating foods and supplementing with omega-3 fatty acids (I will discuss the wonders of omega-3 fatty acids later in the book).

However, lowering triglycerides (something else you can test for with a lipid panel blood test), is very desirable. As a physician, I have witnessed how lower levels of triglycerides improve brain health, memory, heart disease, stroke, and insulin resistance, among other health problems.

Elevated triglycerides typically parallel the increased incidence of obesity and type 2 diabetes.[65] Most often, triglyceride levels increase with the consumption of processed foods, especially highly processed grains and sugars. Lowering triglycerides is best achieved by altering this type of diet and lifestyle, to include eating natural whole foods, and incorporating healthful activities such as time-restricted feeding and exercise.

Take for example a patient, whom we will call John, who came to me with low energy, decreased focus, and was moderately overweight (BMI of 27.4, from a height of 5 feet 8 inches and weight of 180 pounds). He had fasting triglycerides of 300 mg/dl, and HDL of 40, for a TG:HDL ratio of 7.5 (this is considered very elevated).

After changing his diet to primarily a "real/whole" foods diet, largely avoiding processed foods and doing an intermittent fast 5 days a week with the TRF (time-restricted feeding) protocol — where he fasted 16 hours daily, eating during an 8-hour window, 5 days a week — his numbers improved dramatically.

Mind you, he did not count calories, he simply substituted the processed foods he used to eat for real food, changed his eating window from "whenever" to 8 hours a day most days of the week, and added walking to his daily routine. In two months' time, his fasting triglycerides came down to 100 and his HDL came up to 55, for a new TG:HDL ratio of 1.8. Besides this significant improvement in his blood work, he also lost 18 pounds and felt more energized and focused than ever!

Cholesterol is used for all those things we just talked about, and the LDL (the transporter) is required to transport the cholesterol your body needs, distributing it throughout the body at specified locations. Interestingly, longevity studies also show that having higher LDL, especially after age fifty, may contribute to you living longer!

Indeed, in one such recent study from January 2020 by Maihofer et al, this "paradox" was elucidated. They suggested that, "After full adjustment, higher LDL was associated with an increased odds of survival with intact mobility," in their study population of older adults who reached the age of ninety years old.[66]

LDL itself does not necessarily cause heart disease or CAD, because the dangerous type of cholesterol does not travel to the arteries and get deposited there unless it gets oxidized. This oxidation only happens in an inflammatory environment, exacerbated by insulin resistance and the metabolic syndrome. This syndrome is in turn caused by increased blood sugar, obesity, high blood pressure, elevated triglycerides, lack of exercise, consumption of seed oils, and a proinflammatory Western diet rich in highly processed, ultra-refined carbohydrates (grains, flours and sugars).

On the flip side, an anti-inflammatory diet is largely composed of real, whole, natural, unprocessed foods, and lots of antioxidants. Specifically, vegetables and fruit with vitamin E (almonds, avocados, spinach) and the fat-soluble vitamins (D, A, E, K). Some of my favorite antioxidant and vitamin-rich foods are blueberries, strawberries, raspberries, cabbage, kale, artichokes, pecans, and goji berries. They all help decrease the oxidation of the LDL ("bad" cholesterol protein), which means it likely won't stick to the endothelium (lining) of the arteries, and then travel into the wall of the blood vessels, causing the plaques (abnormal cholesterol deposits) of coronary heart disease.

Interestingly, elevated insulin levels (a characteristic of insulin resistance) are not only pro-inflammatory, but increase the production of cholesterol and triglycerides, and are associated with corresponding decreases in the HDL (high-density lipoprotein), or "good" cholesterol.[67] This is literally the perfect storm for setting up the body for chronic disease, and putting yourself at increased risk for heart disease.

And how can we change this?

The key is to keep your insulin low, yet how do we do this?

To sum up, we avoid processed foods (both with refined grains, flours, and sugars — especially high fructose corn syrup), avoid seed oils, remain mindful of the type and amounts of carbohydrates consumed, and time your meals, which we discussed at length in the chapter on Intermittent Fasting.

However, you may get the biggest bang for your buck if you stop snacking, and space out your meals to include an overnight fast of ideally 12–16 hours. Again, remember to discuss any dietary changes, especially if you are on medication, with your healthcare provider.

For now, let us finish strong with the final macronutrient, one of my all-time favorites — powerful protein!

The Power of Protein

What You Need to Know:

- Protein is the basic building block of everything that makes us human
- Daily protein intake is ESSENTIAL as our bodies do not naturally produce it
- Insufficient levels of protein in our bodies lead to a breakdown of our muscles
- A starting point intake of 70 to 140 grams of protein daily is beneficial for most

Protein Power, **ACTIVATE!**

As a kid, I used to watch the cartoon *Wonder Twins*, and go around the house shouting, "Wonder Twin powers, activate!" as I high-fived my brother or sister. Did any of you do that? No...?

Okay. Just thinking of ways to begin the discussion of protein power brought up the memory, and my wanting to share the power of this essential nutrient.

Protein has significant power, and in my humble opinion, is the most powerful and critical of all the macronutrients, because it, quite simply, takes us places. We can move about literally by the power of our protein-filled muscles and connective tissues. And, if we don't pay attention, our muscles may tend to wane as we age — known as age-related sarcopenia — *unless* we do something about it. We will discuss this both here, and in the Movement chapter.

Strap in, locomotion, here we go!

We are what our muscles, joints, skin, and connective tissue are made of — largely protein. Moreover, protein-filled muscle is literally the most metabolically active tissue in the body. Therefore, it is key to understanding and optimizing your metabolism. It is also the basic building block of nearly everything that makes us human, down to the enzymes and the mighty mitochondria we talked about previously. Protein acts, quite frankly, like a basic Lego® brick, linking the vital structural support of the muscles, bones, ligaments, skin, and organs. It is also the key building block from which all our tiny cells and their internal machinery are made.

Protein intake is *essential*. And unlike carbohydrates and fats, it must be derived from our diet, as we have no useful stored form of protein. Yes! I said that right. We must *literally* eat protein daily, for adequate protein intake is key to attaining long-term, overall health.

What I have found in my decades of experience as a physician and health enthusiast is that most people are getting more than enough carbohydrates (*too* many, really) in their diet, but rarely get more than enough protein, especially as we age. This is incredibly important, because our muscles as we get older tend to get smaller and weaker. Taking a proactive approach, by enacting preventative measures like eating daily protein and doing regular resistance training, will aid us in maintaining our musculature and overall health.

> *So, prioritize protein in your diet and in your life!*

Yet before we go into how to ensure we get both adequate protein and the right kind, let us briefly talk about why protein is important in the first place. This essential nutrient is key to health, in numerous ways.

First, we know proteins are literally the building blocks of life, and make up thousands of structures in our bodies. Bones, muscles, skin, and cartilage are primarily made up of proteins, but this is just a small piece of the pie. Literally every cell in the human body contains some type of protein or structure, formed from the basic building blocks of proteins called amino acids. The human body needs protein daily for the growth and repair of its cells, as well as the maintenance of bodily functions, which all occurs through thousands of reactions powered by enzymes, which are also made up of protein.

If you don't get enough protein on a daily basis from your diet, then the body will start to break down its very own muscle in order to supply the adequate protein required to perform the necessary daily functions of the body. This is not only suboptimal, but dangerous to our lifelong health!

As one might imagine, losing muscle mass is not a good thing. Losing muscle not only potentially decreases your overall metabolic rate, but also puts you at risk for deconditioning, which often leads to falls, injuries, and fractures. Moreover, muscle loss contributes to weakness, poor balance, and results in decreased endurance. We need to eat protein daily to not only prevent muscle loss (sarcopenia) but also be able to build it up, and supply the body with the protein it needs to perform essential daily functions, which include a healthy and optimized metabolism.

Unfortunately, studies show that many adults are not getting enough protein in their diet. According to a 2019 study in *The Journal of Nutrition, Health and Aging*, when studying adults over the age of fifty-one, many of them — up to 46% in one group of 3,810 adults — were not receiving the very low minimum requirement of 0.8gm/kg/day of protein intake.[68] In the study, the lower the daily protein intake, the worse the corresponding diet quality was overall too.

The researchers also noted that across all groups, those who had below the daily minimum protein recommendation not only had worse overall nutrition, but also had significantly more functional limitations.[68] This suggests that, despite the increasing popularity of higher protein diets, it is still very common to be protein deficient, especially as we age. Clearly, we still have work to do!

Now that it is clearly established that protein in the diet is essential and required daily, how much do we need? This depends on the individual, but some general guidelines should be considered. Somewhere between 1–2 grams per kilogram of body weight (1.6gm/kg is the minimum used by most fitness experts) is an average baseline that can be adjusted based on your individual goals and circumstances.

For example, someone who weighs 150 pounds (68 kilograms) would need a minimum of 109 grams of protein daily (with a range of 70–140 grams a day) as a starting point. If you wanted to increase your muscle mass, you would consume closer to 2 or 3 grams per kilogram of body weight per day, and if you were simply trying to maintain muscle mass and not increase it, then closer to 1–2 grams/kilograms daily of body weight would be more typical.

Keep in mind your amount of protein intake should certainly be individualized. Furthermore, as we age, we will generally need to increase our protein requirement somewhat, to combat the common condition of sarcopenia. You *can* do this!

Despite the importance of daily protein intake, there exists a large amount of misinformation, especially in the medical and nutrition communities about its consumption. Many still believe that increased protein intake is harmful and damaging to the kidneys, and potentially causes increased cancer risk, which when high-quality prospective data is considered, are both claims that are unfounded.

A 2015 study published in the journal *Advances in Nutrition* found that long-term consumption of protein at 2 g per kg body weight, per day, is safe for healthy adults, and the tolerable upper limit is 3.5 g per kg body weight per day, which is also safe for well-adapted subjects.[69] Although high protein diets have been deemed safe in "normal," healthy individuals, with regular kidney function, it is still recommended to consult your physician prior to starting any new regimen, especially if you have any kidney issues.

Scholarly reviews on increased dietary protein have also shown other positive benefits for our body, such as improvement in metabolism (specifically with increased satiety) and improved thermogenic and glycemic regulation in the body.[70]

Protein intake is definitely something to experiment with as an individual. Start with an initial measurement of how much protein you are getting daily, and go from there. I have found that starting my day with more nutrient and calorically-dense foods, such as healthy proteins and fats, works well for me. I use the mantra *fat and protein first,* and *carbohydrates last,* as carbs are technically nonessential. Instead, they should be eaten towards the end of the meal, and day, to prevent your insulin from spiking first thing in the morning (making you more likely to stop fat burning).

Eating a traditional SAD diet (Standard American Diet) would definitely do this (spike your glucose and corresponding insulin), which is not ideal. The body's innate tendency to be insulin resistant in the morning, (called the *dawn phenomenon*) secondary to the natural morning rise in cortisol, glucose and corresponding insulin, is reason enough to stick to the protein power mantra to start the day!

Another benefit to beginning your day eating a meal with lots of protein, instead of carbohydrates, is that protein tends to be nutrient-dense and much more satiating than a carbohydrate-laden meal. Protein is the most nutritionally dense macronutrient of them all. A healthy, protein-rich meal will keep us fuller, for longer.

Studies show that high protein foods will also increase metabolic rate, which helps with fat burn, weight loss, and energy balance in the body. This concept, that some foods increase metabolic rate more than others, is often referred to as the thermic effect of food (TEF).

Protein, because it takes more energy to digest, actually has the highest energy expenditure. This means that it has a higher metabolic increase from its consumption than fats or carbohydrates. In the *Journal of the American College of Nutrition*, it was proved that protein has a much higher TEF than carbohydrates and fats, up to three times higher, while showing that a high protein diet can also lead to weight loss.[71]

After learning how key protein is to our overall health, the next question that often emerges is how to get protein into our diet? Is there a role for protein powders or supplements? Personally, I strive for appropriate levels of protein and other nutrition goals, with the mindset of *FOOD FIRST.* This includes having healthy protein in every meal and snack I consume. You can then add supplements if you still require more protein after a diet of natural, healthy, well-sourced foods. Yet what are the best go-to, protein-rich foods?

Good news: there are many choices! Both plant and animal-based food options are great. For those that eat both, it is pretty easy to get the required amounts of proteins from many whole real foods.

A selection of animal-based sources:

- Eggs
- Meats (red meat, chicken, turkey, fish, and shellfish)
- Dairy (milk, cheese, Greek yogurt — my personal favorite — cottage cheese, etc.)

A selection of plant-based sources:

- Soy (edamame, tofu, tempeh, miso and natto)
- Nuts (peanuts, almonds, pistachios)
- Beans or legumes (lentils, soybeans, kidney beans, chickpeas)
- Seeds (pumpkin, flax, sunflower, chia)
- Grains (quinoa, millet, barley, spelt, oats)
- Vegetables (broccoli, Brussels sprouts, asparagus)

Remember, though, neither of these are exhaustive lists.

If you still can't get enough protein from your diet, then a protein supplement is a reasonable option, which can be obtained from both plant and animal sources. When choosing a supplement, always keep in mind the quality of its source, that it comes from a reputable brand, and that it is third-party validated for both quality, purity and potency. These are basic rules of thumb to keep in mind with *any* supplementation.

Human protein is more similar to the animal proteins which may be found in our diet. Animal proteins tend to be "complete" proteins (they typically contain all nine of the essential amino acids which are required of any healthy diet). Therefore, these animal proteins tend to have a higher PDCAA quality and digestibility score than their plant-based counterparts, as they are more similar to the proteins in the human body. The PDCAA is the "Protein Digestibility Corrected Amino Acid Score." This score evaluates protein quality, by comparing the food's amino acid composition to what our bodies can normally use.

Let us compare milk and quinoa. Milk and red meat typically have a PDCAA score near 100% digestibility, whereas quinoa has a lower value of 70% digestibility. This is in general terms, and does not take into consideration if someone may be lactose intolerant, for example. Pea protein is usually in the 70% range, while protein from lentils and peanuts is lower, in the 50% range.

What this means is that someone would need to consume a larger volume of quinoa in order to get the same amount of protein you would get from a grass-fed steak, ounce per ounce, as red meat is more nutrient dense. Plant protein tends to be less nutritionally dense, and comes with additional carbohydrates. No matter your choice, pay attention to the sourcing of the product, as it is better for your overall health to consume organic, non-GMO, pesticide-free, antibiotic-free, hormone-free, and well-sourced plant or animal protein.

For supplementing animal protein, interestingly enough, "whey isolate" would be a good first choice. It is largely devoid of casein and lactose, which is the component of milk to which most have allergies or intolerances. So, use high quality well sourced whey isolate as a protein source if you can have animal protein in your diet.

As far as plant-based protein supplements go, soy and pea protein are typically regarded as the only complete proteins of those readily available from plants. I lean towards pea over soy, as sourcing tends to be better with pea protein. If you are not able to consume adequate plant protein from soy in the form of tofu, tempeh, or edamame, a plant-based protein supplement with soy protein, pea protein, or even rice protein, can be a great option. Try to get organic, non-GMO if at all possible when sourcing plant proteins.

Indeed, it is certainly possible to get good quality plant-based protein from your diet, including protein with essential amino acids. To ensure that you do, try several of these plant-based proteins together. Mix it up! Mix your pea with your rice protein. This is a great way to ensure all nine of the essential amino acid profiles are met. Because remember, many plant proteins are not complete.

Yet this is not a push towards being either primarily plant or animal-based in your diet — either can achieve great health. I am simply imparting information to help guide your selections of the best nutrients, from both plant and animal kingdoms.

Personally, I aim to consume both high-quality plant and animal protein, as they come with different corresponding nutrient profiles. Myself, I enjoy digging into a well-seasoned, juicy steak, along with a side of Brussel sprouts, and well-seasoned organic edamame or miso soup. Can you tell I love a meal from a great Japanese steak house with all of the above? And if you are ever in Hawaii, I can give you some great recommendations.

You will soon understand why exercise is such a key ingredient to overall health and weight management, in the Movement chapter. Yet just to further highlight the importance of protein here, it is definitely needed in a workout routine. In order to fully optimize our exercise experience, we need to make sure we are getting adequate protein in the diet. Fortunately, this is not difficult to get started.

First, you must *measure* it! A simple way to do this is to use an app like MyFitnessPal or MyPlate, and start adding the foods you are eating, just to get a baseline of your typical daily protein intake, and then go from there. This is what I did, and found that I was not getting the amount of protein I thought I was from my diet, and have therefore added more dietary protein, and also supplementation, to achieve my protein goals.

Remember to get high-quality proteins from fresh, real, natural, and whole foods, whether from plants, animals, or both, and stick with the mantra: *food first*. If you still need more protein, a high-quality supplement may be a good choice to get your 1–3g/kg of body weight in protein each day. The benefits are seemingly endless!

The benefits of protein and muscle health go far beyond weight loss and simply building muscle tissue. It can help improve brain health, metabolic health, and even help you age better by preventing sarcopenia. So, are you now ready to make sure your daily foods have sufficient protein?

Some of you may ask, "What about those that say protein is not good for you, or that it causes decreased longevity? What about the activation of that thing called mTOR? Can you speak to that?"

Of course, I thought you would never ask!

Yet I will also do so concisely, as entire books could be written on this topic alone.

First of all, similar to studies on saturated fat which were mentioned earlier in the book, I could not find a single high-quality, randomized controlled trial (RCT) on how increased protein in the diet causes reduced longevity or early death. In fact, when I researched this, what I did find was the exact opposite! I found that RCTs evaluating a high protein diet actually showed a mortality benefit, not an earlier death.

Negative reviews on protein typically use low-quality epidemiological studies, or even rat models. For example, a recent 2020 review of 31 different high-quality RCT studies reported in the *British Medical Journal* (a very prestigious, trusted, high-quality, and peer-reviewed medical journal) shared that high protein diets actually improve mortality, instead of worsening it. This included high protein diets from both plant *and* animal sources.[72]

So why have some in the media and purported longevity influencers reported supposed adverse effects or concerns of protein, when referring to something called mTOR? Well, let's address this.

To begin with, mTOR is the "mammalian target of rapamycin," which is an enzyme complex responsible for cellular growth, and in particular, muscle cell growth. This enzyme complex is somewhat generic in nature, and is turned on in the body with nearly any kind of cellular growth that is considered "good growth," like growing muscle tissue as a result of resistance training or increased protein in the diet. "Bad growth" would be a cancerous tumor, or the often "undesired growth" of fat or adipose tissue.

This mTOR concept is not cut and dry; mTOR activation is general and somewhat indiscriminate. We need it turned on and in use for normal body functions, like muscle growth, but we would also benefit from it being turned off for periods of time (intermittent fasting).

We can look at this as a case of the classic Goldilocks phenomenon: too little mTOR activity may result in protein deficiency, even sarcopenia, and poor nutrition and health, yet too much mTOR activity could lead to obesity and cancer. Therefore, we want to get the "right amount" of mTOR activity, as we cannot simply turn it off exclusively in the hopes of increased longevity, and still expect to maintain essential vital functions.

These mTOR pathways, how they are turned on and off during growth, and their role in metabolism and disease, are well described in a review article from 2017 in the scientific journal *Cell*.[73] Here, the various signals that turn mTOR activity on and off were discussed in relation to the possible promotion of longevity, as well as the significant limitations of cancer and other disease treatments.

Unfortunately, most of the data on this topic comes from other simpler organisms such as fruit flies, yeast, and mice. A relative paucity of relevant human data exists, though it certainly remains an area of active research and could likely provide significant benefits in the future.

To summarize, mTOR activity, as a result of eating protein, should not be a significant concern if you are trying to build muscle and increase your health and fitness. Aim to source the best quality foods as a part of your healthy intake of protein. What should be a forefront concern is having elevated levels of insulin, and correspondingly mTOR, by continuously snacking and eating low-quality, calorically dense and nutrient-poor foods.

For now, focus on eating **real, whole, natural**, and largely **unprocessed** foods that are well-sourced. *Time* your meals appropriately, and minimize your snacking, to maximize your benefits. Find out how much protein your body needs, and start to consume the appropriate amount daily. This will allow you to begin your journey towards greater muscle, heart, brain, and total body health.

The bottom line, however, is that I wouldn't worry about mTOR — as long as you are optimizing the health principles taught in this book!

CHAPTER 4

What's in Your Kitchen?

> *"The doctor of the future will no longer treat the human frame with drugs, but rather will cure and prevent disease with nutrition."*
> –Thomas Edison

As we have discussed, *food is medicine*. It is the *most* important and *frequent* medicine we can take. Food can be used to not only fuel our bodies, but to energize and empower us for both today's, and a lifetime's, worth of optimized health, performance, and enjoyment!

Food can and should be enjoyed!

Unfortunately, in the Western world, we have essentially limited ourselves to only a few primary sources, which make up the majority of our diet. In fact, although there are more than 200,000 edible species of plants, over fifty percent of our caloric intake as humans is made up of only three – corn, wheat and rice.

So even though we may need to subtract a few less healthful items from our pantry, which will be explained below, we also have much more to *add*, rather than subtract, within the big picture! Remember, *diversity* is the *spice* of life — for our health, happiness, and palate!

Let's get started!

The Pantry Purge

Now that we have discussed each of the macros, you will have a good idea of what to *add* to your diet (there are so many new, exciting, and tasty whole foods, both fresh, raw, and even fermented). Still, you are probably wondering about the things that we need to subtract — those that are unhealthy. You need not fret, however, as it is really quite simple.

Let's first take a moment to look at this in a little more detail, and you will then be ready to do the "pantry purge" activity. In the future, most of this will be done at the grocery store, and you won't have to dump things from your pantry because you will have already made the correct healthy choices at your local market or grocery store.

Remember, if you don't want to be tempted to eat certain highly processed "junk foods," never allow them into your cart or basket at the grocery store in the first place! A good rule of thumb at the grocery store is to do most of your shopping on the perimeter of the store, where the fresh vegetables, fruits, and proteins are located, and less in the center of the store, which is largely where the processed foods are located. Focus on this, and you will be off to a great start!

To help you with *optimizing* your *macros*, and stop consuming foods that may break your metabolism, let us do a quick **pantry purge** activity. Note, if you don't want to put the items you already have in the trash, and they are unopened and have not expired, you can also consider donating them to a local food pantry.

> *Remember:*
> *The nature and quality of your food*
> *is everything.*

What to Toss

Use the Five Ingredient Rule — any items that contain more than five ingredients, especially those you are not familiar with or sound like they belong in a chemistry lab, ought to be considered for discarding.

Also, discard those items which have mystery chemicals, or that are potentially harmful. Think of any artificial color, flavor, or additive, and any chemicals you don't recognize. Remember, what is in your pantry should be **food**, *not* anything that sounds like it should be in a chemistry lab.

You should be able to recognize the ingredients, and they should be from real foods. If not, consider tossing them out! In the future, this will get a lot easier, as most of these unhealthy items will not end up in your pantry at all, because you will apply this **five ingredient rule**, right at the grocery store!

Check the packaging — If there is BPA in the lining of the can or in plastic packaging, **toss it!**

Toss anything over 1-2 years old or beyond expiration; also toss flour or other baking goods not in an airtight container (beware of the weevils).

Toss open/unused items, or those with damaged packaging. Then, **most importantly**, start **reading the labels**, and apply the tools on the next page.

What to Avoid

- **Artificial colors and sweeteners***
- **HFCS (high fructose corn syrup)** or corn syrup, as these are notorious for causing high triglycerides, fatty liver, insulin resistance and contributing to the leading cause of non alcoholic fatty liver disease which is now the most common cause for liver transplant and is completely preventable!
- **Seed oils** and hydrogenated oils or trans fats ("fake fats")**: though hydrogenated oils and partially hydrogenated oils are known to be unsafe and deemed as such by the FDA in 2015, they are still commonly found in processed foods, but you won't know unless you read the label.
- **MSG, nitrates and nitrites, carrageenan, sodium benzoate, trans fat (hydrogenated oils and spreads), and other unfamiliar chemicals like the azodicarbonamide in yoga mats, and some breads or butylated hydroxytoluene (BHT) used in various foods as a preservative.**
- **Most chips and crackers** (apply the above rules here).
- **Most salad dressings** (see above criteria and especially avoid those with the seed oils).
- **Most cereals and granolas** (follow ingredients rules above).
- **Most mayos, sauces, and spreads** (unless they pass the ingredient rules above).
- **Highly processed sugars, carbohydrates, and flours.**

*Aim to have natural sweeteners (monk fruit, stevia, etc.) over highly processed ones such as high-fructose corn syrup (HFCS), processed sugars like brown rice syrup, corn syrup, dextrose, maltose and non-nutritive sweeteners like sucralose (Splenda), saccharin (SweetNLow), acesulfame-k (Sweet One, Sunnett), or neotame, aspartame (NutraSweet) — look on the ingredients list of both your pantry foods and your vitamins/supplements, too. You may be surprised at what you will find in those "healthy" multivitamins and snack bars, for example.

Avoid the *seed oils* which are canola, corn, cottonseed, sunflower, ricebran, grapeseed, safflower, soy and soybean, and hydrogenated oils of all kinds. These are all highly processed industrialized oils which are heavily damaged in the processing with extreme heat, high pressures, exposure to harsh chemicals like toluene and other solvents to deodorize and bleach them to hide their rancid heavily oxidized nature. They are also very PUFA rich (polyunsaturated fatty acids), **cause inflammation, and may cause or contribute to many adverse health conditions. The *healthy* oils *to replace them with* are: pure extra virgin olive, avocado, coconut or MCT oil, unrefined palm, Macadamia nut, and almond oil, as well as cocoa butter or natural fats such as butter, ghee, tallow, and lard, as long as these are well-sourced, for example from grass-fed pasture-raised animals. Think of the natural oils we have been using for millenia which essentially do not require any processing other than simple pressing or squeezing such as with the oil from olives, avocados or coconuts. Try to get products with these healthier oils that are whole or minimally processed (better if "pressed" and not "refined," as refined means more industrial processing.)

Bottom line is, there are only a few general categories of foods to avoid and many more to add to our diet, more than two thousand of them! "Eat the Rainbow," is the mantra I often use as a reminder of the myriad of colorful healthy whole foods that are available to us. Variety and diversity are the spice of life for our palate, planet and overall health!

The simple way I remember those few foods to avoid is by an easy threesome, I affectionately call the "Evil Triad." These are the highly processed **grains/flours, sugars, and seed oils**. When you simply avoid these three main ingredients, the highly processed chemicals and ingredients above, and replace them with real whole foods, the difference will be palpable and set you on the path toward optimal health.

To Supplement or Not to Supplement?
That is the Question!

> *"You can trace every sickness, every disease, and every ailment to a mineral deficiency."*
>
> - **Dr. Linus Pauling, two-time Nobel Prize winner**

In a perfect world *without* pollution, stress, chemical exposures from pesticides, herbicides, plastics, or EMF (electric and magnetic field) exposure, and *with* perfectly natural foods grown from the richest soils, supplementation likely would not be necessary. On this planet we call Earth — an awesome place by the way, though far from perfect — these conditions don't currently exist. Thus, supplementation is not only helpful for optimal health, but to some degree necessary.

It has been known for years that our soils are rapidly becoming deficient in many nutrients. And given the industrialized agricultural techniques that have been employed over the last several centuries (mono-crop agriculture, machine-based tilling, widespread pesticide use, etc.), this is no surprise.

A very interesting senate report from 1936 reported on this topic, and discussed the corresponding work by a physician named Dr. Charles Northern. Dr. Northern became so passionate about the importance of healthy soil being paramount to human health that he largely left his medical practice to develop techniques for improving soil health, in order to thereby improve human health.

In the 1936 report, it was said of Dr. Northern, "This quiet, unbally-hooed pioneer and genius in the field of nutrition demonstrates that countless human ills stem from the fact that the impoverished soil of America no longer provides plant foods with the mineral elements essential to human nourishment and health! To overcome this alarming condition, he doctors sick soils and, by seeming miracles, raises truly healthy and health-giving fruits and vegetables."[74]

Dr. Northern was on point with his approach, and ahead of his time. **Healthy people come from healthy food, which comes from healthy soil.** Unfortunately, his honorable mission largely fell upon deaf ears in the U.S. Senate, and though it has been known for nearly a century that our soils are depleted of many minerals and nutrients, very little has been done about it. This is thus an even greater reason for us to seek the highest quality, best-sourced food available.

Besides the fact that most of our food is lacking sufficient levels of vitamins and minerals, many of us also eat processed foods (think anything in a bag or box with a bar code or a label). These foods may certainly be calorie-rich, but are often very nutrient-poor. In fact, most of the processed foods we are familiar with (nearly all processed and packaged snack food, bread, pasta, cereals, etc.) are basically devoid of any appreciable amount of nutrients. Just think about it, why else would they have to be "fortified?" This is a true double whammy!

Not only are processed foods making us fat (containing highly inflammatory ingredients with flours, sugars, and seed oils), they have next to nothing as far as true nutritional value. I believe this is a grave problem in our society — we are calorically overfed with processed foods, and at the same time seriously undernourished. One might say we are quite literally starving for nutrients, in a sea of plenty.

It has been suggested that part of our overfed diet may be due to an insatiable craving for more nutrients, since most of the processed food we consume is devoid of them. Our body seeks more and more calories, in an attempt to fill its nutrient void. Therefore, filling our vitamin and mineral gaps with higher quality foods and appropriate supplements may be crucial to meeting our health and nutrient needs, and will likely lead to more energy, less cravings, vitality, and better health.

Speaking to this need for supplementation, a well-known and respected physician who has done a lot of work in this area over the years, Dr. Mark Hyman, has shared a pearl of knowledge that is certainly worth mentioning.

He suggests:

"Even with a perfect diet, the combination of many things — including our depleted soils, the storage and transportation of our food, genetic alterations of traditional heirloom species, and the increased stress and nutritional demands resulting from a toxic environment – make it impossible for us to get the vitamins and minerals we need solely from the foods we eat."[75]

This is strong language, stating that it is not only difficult but *impossible* to get all the necessary vitamins and minerals we need, solely from food. I'd add, however, that this doesn't mean we shouldn't try. *Food first* has and always will be my mantra, then supplement to fill in the gaps, as needed.

I realize it may be easier to simply take a pill (be it medication or supplement) for X, Y, or Z health issues or deficiencies. But I submit, it is absolutely necessary that we treat our *food* truly as *medicine* — striving to get the most out of a natural, healthy, unprocessed, and well-sourced whole foods diet.

Food honestly is the best and most frequent medicine we can give to ourselves — we deserve this! And, if we optimize it, we will profoundly profit both in our enjoyment of many delicious and nutritious natural whole foods, and reap their huge health benefits.

Therefore, as I mentioned previously, I use the *food first* mantra, and start by building my diet with vitamin and mineral-rich, fresh, and unprocessed natural, real whole foods (making up the difference with supplementation). Remember, supplements should really be treated as their name suggests: supplemental, and should come after a natural, real, well-sourced whole foods diet to fill in the gaps.

When getting the most out of our diet, we should carefully choose our foods from those best sourced and of the highest quality available in our local markets, while realizing there *may* be some deficits. Yet it is important to remember that deficits are common, and thoughtful supplementation can help fill in the gaps.

But in no way should supplements take the place of a healthy, natural, high-quality, and well-sourced real food diet. In the same way that NO amount of exercise can ever make up for a crappy diet — NO amount of supplementation can either.

> *Choose FOOD FIRST,*
> *then fill in the gaps.*

Now we have accepted that supplementation may be necessary, what does the average person need? I'll try to keep to the point here, because a lengthy supplement discussion is far beyond the scope of this chapter, and indeed this book. I'd also like you to discuss your nutrition, diet, and supplement needs with your personal healthcare or nutrition provider, to tailor a plan that fits you. To give you a basic foundation, however, I want to provide a short list of the "biggest bang for your buck" supplements from which most of us can benefit right away.

Keep in mind first that the *quality* of the supplement matters. Try to look for those that are well-sourced supplements, preferably coming from real food (plants such as vegetables or fruits, and well-sourced animal products) whenever possible. These well-sourced supplements that come from real living organisms, plants, and animals, are going to be better utilized by the body than a synthetic any day of the week.

Many top-selling vitamins and supplements are synthetically bulk processed in similar chemical labs that many pharmaceutical companies use. For example, *Centrum* is made by the pharmaceutical company Pfizer. Arguably the most popular kids vitamin, *Flintstone*, and the well-known vitamin for adults *One a Day*, come from the Bayer pharmaceutical company. Another top seller, *Theragran-M*, formerly owned by Bristol Myers Squibb, was recently acquired by Walgreens.

Now, I am not saying that these large pharmaceutical companies are not capable of making quality vitamins — you be the judge. Just take a look at the labels. For example, all of the brand names just mentioned use a laboratory-derived folate in their multivitamin — the synthetic form of folic acid, not the bioavailable form of methyl-folate.

In addition, many popular children's vitamins tend to use sugars like glucose, fructose, and even synthetic artificial sweeteners like sucralose, among other unnatural ingredients. The bottom line: with supplements, like with food, **you need to read the label**. Both quality and sourcing of the ingredients used matter just as much as they do with food, so don't forget to do this — you may be surprised by what you find.

Beyond passing the ingredients and label test, you must also make sure the supplement manufacturers you choose employ good manufacturing practices (GMPs). Make sure the products are third-party validated and tested for quality, purity, potency, and lack of contaminants (some labels may include USP [the U.S. Pharmacopeial Convention] or NSF International certification), or you may look for verification through websites such as Labdoor.com and Consumerlabs.com.

Do a little research on the company, read the label, and do not buy the first thing that pops up on Amazon, social media, or anywhere else on the internet. I've found many forms of sugar and artificial colors or sweeteners present in many vitamins, both children and adult versions. So, once more from the rooftops, **read the labels!** Don't assume that just because you bought it from a vitamin store or website that it is of good quality and sourced well.

Instead look for supplements that are organic, non-GMO, gluten-free, without additives, fillers, artificial colors or sweeteners, flavors, or preservatives and preferably sourced in a country or location you are familiar with and trust.

And with that being said, let's now dive into some of my favorite supplements that pack the most punch!

Multivitamins

A good multivitamin is really the cornerstone of a solid supplement regimen. Adding an MVM (multivitamin/mineral) helps address any possible nutritional gaps we may experience. For most of us, the potential benefits will likely outweigh the low risk of this simple intervention.[76] This is a relatively low-cost, low-risk method of filling in your vitamin and mineral gaps.

As with foods, supplements are not all created equal. Again, please remember to read the label! Personally, I try to pick a multivitamin that uses the most bioavailable form of nutrients. This should be a no-brainer: why wouldn't you pick the one that closely resembles the form of vitamin or mineral your body actually uses, right? Though this may seem like common sense, most doctors do not pay attention to this. Case in point: folate.

Your multivitamin should contain folate, because not only does it help prevent neural tube defects while promoting fetal health (OBGYNs recommend it), it may also help decrease the risk of heart disease, cancer, and other chronic diseases. Folate is involved in the homocysteine metabolic pathway. A deficiency of folate and/or vitamin B12, both of which act as cofactors in the breakdown of homocysteine, can thus lead to increased homocysteine. This is a risk factor for vascular disease and blood clots, predisposing one to heart attack, stroke, and pulmonary embolism (blood clot in the lungs).

Folate, rather than folic acid (often prescribed), is thus preferable.

I use a fully methylated form, L-methylfolate, which is generally more useful and bioavailable for most people. This is especially important to consider given many people have one of the several MTHFR (methylenetetrahydrofolate reductase) genetic mutations or variants (these are surprisingly common). Therefore, they may not be able to process the synthetic folic acid well.

In these cases of MTHFR genetic mutations or variants (which affect a significant portion of the population), supplementing with 5-methylfolate (shortened from 5-methyltetrahydrofolate) can then increase the active folate, and replete the deficiency in the body. On the other hand, using the commonly prescribed multivitamin containing folic acid in this case would unlikely replace the deficit.[77]

A lengthy discussion of the MTHFR genetic mutations/variants is beyond the scope of the book, but having your health care provider test for the most common ones is prudent, as these can be something that surprisingly affects many people. Just remember, having methylated folate in your multivitamin, like L-methylfolate (not folic acid), is a good place to start. Look for it on the labels!

I also look for a multivitamin that contains the active bioavailable form of Vitamin B12, or methylcobalamin. Vitamin B12 is essential for healthy nerve and blood cells,

DNA synthesis, and repair, as well as homocysteine pathway health, as discussed.

Vitamin B12 deficiency is actually pretty common. In my practice, I've found that many people unknowingly are low or even deficient in it. My uncle, for example, who has a great whole foods diet and is generally in good health, started to have neurologic symptoms: numbness in his feet and legs primarily, as well as difficulty with balance and walking. Soon after identifying the symptoms, we discovered he had a vitamin B12 deficiency, as he was largely eating a vegan diet. Fortunately, his symptoms were completely resolved after restoring his vitamin B12.

Groups of people especially at risk for low B12 and/or deficiency are vegetarians and vegans, the elderly, those with gut issues (especially malabsorption or those on chronic acid-reducing medications), and alcohol dependency.[78] Having your health care provider check your vitamin B12 level is a great idea, while I advise you to get checked for homocysteine levels as well. If a multivitamin is needed, choose the active bioavailable natural form, methylcobalamin!

Looking for the presence of selenium and zinc in your multivitamin is also an adviseable approach. Because our bodies do not naturally produce and store it like it does sugars and fats, we need to get zinc from our food and supplements. Zinc is useful for numerous things, as it is a cofactor in hundreds of reactions in the body.

It is important for immune function, decreasing inflammation, its antioxidant properties, healthy skin, eye health, wound healing, DNA and protein production, and numerous other enzymatic functions. During the pandemic, it also received news coverage for its benefits in immune function, as well as its role in taste and smell.[205] It may also improve testosterone levels in those with low zinc levels.[79] Zinc optimization is essential, and can be found in a great multivitamin.

Selenium is also an essential mineral, with many important health benefits, but is often lacking in many diets. It is a very powerful antioxidant that supports our metabolism and thyroid function, and may reduce the risks of cancer, heart disease, and cognitive decline. Many people are deficient in selenium — unless you are eating a couple of Brazil nuts daily (these are an excellent source), you may want to have your primary physician check you for deficiency.

In addition to these essential nutrients, I generally look for a multivitamin that also contains 100% of the U.S. RDA (Recommended Dietary Allowances) of Vitamins C, D, E, A, K (containing both K1 and K2 is a plus), and the B vitamins (thiamine, riboflavin, niacin, pantothenic acid, pyridoxine, and biotin). If your multivitamin-mineral supplement contains the U.S. RDA of chromium (important for decreasing insulin resistance and for blood sugar balance), manganese, and copper, that's an additional bonus.

And if you can find a multivitamin that has all of these essentials, you will be in extremely good shape!

Vitamin D

Vitamin D has long been one of my favorite vitamins, for many reasons. One of the things I love most about it is, if you live in a place where you can get adequate sunshine without getting burned, you can get it for FREE! Out in the sunshine, you can optimize your vitamin D in as little as 10–15 minutes a day.

Going outside also has the bonus of fresh air, and Vitamin "N" (nature), as I like to call it, and can dramatically positively affect your mood and brain health. The benefits of nature are numerous and far-reaching, so during your 15 minutes of outside time while breathing fresh air and soaking in Vitamin D, try to access some of them.

As I previously mentioned, vitamin D has also received increased press in light of the recent pandemic, due to its significant effects in boosting immune health. It is technically a fat-soluble vitamin that acts more like a hormone. Thus, it has a myriad of functions.

More than 50% of the human population have insufficient vitamin D, and here in the U.S. and farther north, it is likely more than 70%. Those with more natural melanin in their skin, diabetes, who are obese, have a poor health status, and who smoke have an increased risk of being deficient.[80]

Yet it is not only adults who are deficient. Recently reported in the scientific journal *Pediatrics*, up to 70% of children are also low in this crucial vitamin.[81] Lower levels of Vitamin D have also been linked to increased risk of infection (including COVID-19), cardiovascular disease, cancer, and even depression.[82, 83, 84]

Vitamin D is crucial for hundreds of reactions in the body, and has been linked to the regulation of between 100-1250 genes![85] If you are deficient, simply taking the small amount contained in your multivitamin may not be enough to replenish it. As I mentioned, then, my goal first and foremost is to get mine from daily sun exposure, depending on the season and where I am in the world. I also try to eat vitamin D-rich foods (fatty, fresh, and wild-caught fish [like ahi or tuna], eggs, and yogurt). In the winter I often need to supplement as well. In choosing my supplements, I make sure to use the active form, vitamin D3, and check my levels every 2 months or so.

Checking your 25-hydroxy vitamin D level is a good start (shoot for a level above 50 ng/ml). Make sure you supplement with the active form, vitamin D3, or cholecalciferol, and look for a maintenance dose of around 2000 IU (international units) daily, which is equivalent to 50 mcg (micrograms). Please note that you may need a much higher dose (from 5000–10,000 IU daily) to get your levels to a healthy number if you have been deficient for 2–3 months.

It's a great idea to check your current 25-hydroxy vitamin D levels for a reference point, and then again in 2 months after supplementing, to see where you are, and adjust accordingly with the help of your provider. Not only will repleting your vitamin D help your immune function, but also likely elevate your mood, decrease insulin resistance, and reduce your risk of many chronic inflammatory diseases such as heart disease, autoimmune diseases like multiple sclerosis, and even cancer.

Furthermore, you might notice that replenishing your vitamin D may even help you lose weight! In a double-blind prospective trial reported in the *International Journal of Preventive Medicine*, they found that after six weeks of vitamin D supplementation in the intervention group, they had significant weight loss, in addition to significant decreases in waist and hip circumference and BMI, compared to the control group without the supplemental Vitamin D.[86]

Vitamin D for the win, AGAIN!

Magnesium

Magnesium is my favorite mineral. It is both mighty and magnificent in so many ways. It does so much in the body (it is involved in over 600 reactions),[87] and is important for optimal body and brain health. In fact, it is *necessary* to make the energy, or ATP, in our body every moment we are alive, which is vital to metabolism and life![88] Without magnesium, we would literally be devoid of energy, and die!

Sadly, according to the medical journal *American Family Physician*, up to 75 percent of us are not getting the recommended amount in our daily diet.[89] Also, it is often not included in adequate amounts in a multivitamin, because the amount we need can only fit into a bulky pill (it would make for a super large multivitamin tablet or capsule). As a result, I generally encourage people to take a separate magnesium supplement.

Low magnesium intake has been linked to not only muscle and bone problems, but also increased risk of depression and mood/anxiety problems, poor sleep, elevated blood pressure, low energy (not surprising given its crucial importance in making ATP), diabetes, and insulin resistance, as well as irregular heartbeat and asthma progression.

Magnesium is easy to replenish with supplementation. Some foods do contain magnesium, like certain nuts and seeds (especially almonds, pumpkin seeds, and peanuts), though you would have to consume about 1/2 to 3/4 of a pound daily to get the necessary amount — that is a lot of nuts! I love nuts, but I am not going to eat that many each day, so I supplement daily with magnesium.

Now, I urge you not to not grab the least expensive, poorly absorbed forms, such as magnesium oxide, magnesium gluconate, magnesium carbonate, and magnesium sulfate. They tend to go right through the gastrointestinal tract, causing diarrhea, rather than replenishing your stores. Magnesium sulfate, or Epsom salt, is often used in bathwater to soothe the muscles, but is not awesome as an oral supplement, as it has both an unpleasant taste and smell, is poorly absorbed, and often causes diarrhea.

There are many great forms, however, that are highly recommendable. These include magnesium threonate (my personal favorite, as it enters the brain more easily by crossing the brain-blood barrier, and can help with headaches, mood, and sleep), magnesium glycinate (also absorbed well from the GI tract, and tends to have fewer side effects of diarrhea), magnesium orotate (may improve heart function), magnesium citrate (often used to help with constipation), magnesium lactate (well absorbed and gentler on the GI tract), and magnesium malate (easily absorbed and has been used with fibromyalgia).

This may seem like a lot to remember, so if you'd rather have just one or two choices, I'd stick to either magnesium glycinate or magnesium threonate; both are easily absorbed, and work well from my experience.

Omega-3s (EPA And DHA)

Though many of us have heard of the tremendous heart and brain health benefits of Omega-3, Americans do not get enough of it in our diet to reap the benefits, according to a study in *Nutrition Journal*.[90] Given this, we may need additional supplementation.

Omega-3 fatty acids, specifically EPA (eicosapentaenoic acid) and DHA (docosahexaenoic acid), promote eye and brain health. Additional benefits include: helping with depressive disorders such as anxiety and ADHD, decreasing the risk of Alzheimer's disease, inflammation, as well as improving joint and skin health, immunity, sport performance, and cardiovascular health.[90, 91, 92, 93, 94] With all of these benefits, why are we not taking advantage?

Most Americans do not eat the recommended two meals a week containing fatty fish — anchovies, mackerel, salmon, sardines, herring, trout, tuna, caviar, and oysters. I love fish, but often find it difficult to get those that are well-sourced, wild-caught, low mercury-containing, so I also supplement. Yet, again, when possible my mantra is food first, as both DHA and EPA are found in fatty fish. The smaller fish such as anchovies and sardines tend to be the lowest in potential mercury toxicity and also the fish eggs (roe of which caviar is just one subtype and delicacy of the sturgeon variety) tend to also have significant omega-3 with less mercury risk. Fish roe is becoming more common and available too.

In plants, the omega-3 alpha-linolenic acid (ALA) is present in: flaxseed, chia, hemp, soybeans, and walnuts. However, these are not the best source for bioavailable Omega-3s, and certainly not as good as a fish source. The reason is that EPA and DHA are not generally found in plants, so the plant ALA must then be *converted* to EPA and DHA, in a lengthy biochemical process inside the body. And this process only occurs 1–10% of the time, making it terribly inefficient.[95, 96]

If you are unable to eat fish at least twice a week, you likely will need to supplement with some form of fish oil containing EPA and DHA. Fortunately, these supplements are abundant and readily available, just remember to apply the guidelines mentioned previously to obtain the best ones, derived from quality, well-sourced, whole food. Typically taking 1000 to 2000 mg of the combo (EPA/DHA) once or twice a day is a good place to start. If you prefer a vegan source, the algae-derived ones tend to be superior to those only containing ALA.

So, that's the wrap for my short-listed, high-powered combo of supplements that I take after starting with *real foods first*. I fill in the gaps with the above essentials, which in totality has served me, my family, and many others well. Be sure to discuss your new regimen with your healthcare and nutrition providers, and tailor a plan that fits your needs.

Remember, this is not a prescription to replace a solid, well-sourced, real foods diet. This is primordial, because food truly is medicine. NO amount of supplements can cancel out the effects of a crappy diet. NONE. Focus on a high-quality, natural, real foods diet, then fill in the gaps with high-impact supplements as needed. I know that for me, I am glad I did, and recommend you take a look at your potential supplement needs as well!

CHAPTER 5

Sleep it Off

> *"Sleep is the golden chain that ties health and our bodies together."*
> -   **Thomas Dekker**

No, I am not talking about the hangover you may want to sleep off. I'm talking about *losing weight naturally*, optimizing your health and longevity by improving your sleep! This one action may do more for your health and lifespan than anything else, and it's completely FREE! It is a powerful and simple activity that has changed numerous lives — including mine. I've experienced short and long-term results, making this a true game-changer.

I'll be honest, this was not always something I appreciated or understood. It has been quite the opposite in my case. Throughout my twelve years of medical training, sleep was often looked upon as a sign of weakness. Medical training in the 1990s involved a "beat you down" kind of mentality — the one who stayed awake the longest or worked the most consecutive hours or days got the proverbial "badge of honor." It's certainly not something I am proud of having participated in as a physician, but I learned much on account of it. Yet soon after, I committed myself to NOT repeating that foolish practice of disregarding the power and benefits of adequate quality sleep.

In that environment, I cultivated the attitude of "I'll sleep when I'm dead." Anyone a fan of the rock group *The Cure*? They recorded a song called "Sleep When I'm Dead" that topped the singles charts of their *4:13 Dream* album in 2008, which stamped my belief in not wasting too much time sleeping that I began in college, and continued throughout medical school and residency training. Afterward, while working at a community hospital for several years, I still fostered this notion that sleep is not a high priority and often a waste of time, at least to some degree. There was just too much I wanted to do: work 100 hours a week, make time for my wife and kids, and surf. I did all that, but it definitely did not leave much time for sleep.

Why do I mention this? Well, for two reasons. Not only did I love the band *The Cure* as a youth in the 1980s, but this notion of sleep being a weakness and an activity overachievers would not waste much time doing was pervasive in my medical training. I remember so vividly my medical school neurology professor giving a lecture on exactly that — sleep — and how it was overrated. He taught that although we spend nearly one-third of our lives in bed, there was no concrete science showing why it was needed.

A lot of data collected in the last several decades has changed our collective understanding of sleep and its health benefits. Sleep is a simple activity that can be optimized to levels that allow for positive dividends in our overall health and lifespan. More importantly, it lends rewards to our day-to-day enjoyment of life. Just ask my wife how pleasant I was during my endless hours of medical training focused around very little sleep. I was definitely not always great to be around, and could frequently be described as cranky or grouchy. It was all because my average sleep time was between 4–6 hours a night. At the time, I prided myself on that schedule. That is until I began to better understand the power of sleep.

However, you do not, and should not, have to suffer through decades of sleep deprivation like I did. Realizing that life can be better, healthier, and happier with optimized sleep will save you a myriad of health problems later. The good news is science has now amassed a vast amount of knowledge on this topic in recent years. The rationale behind why we need sleep in the first place, its numerous corresponding benefits, and how sleep can be optimized for prime health, are all factors that can be applied to our action plan for long-term weight loss.

For years it has been known that sleep is necessary for cognitive function. We long appreciated that if one did not get any sleep or enough sleep, they could not perform certain tasks as effectively, which increased their risk of developing certain health issues. Yet we still did not truly understand from a physiological perspective why sleep was necessary. It was unclear what actually occurs in our bodies during sleep that makes it such a valuable aspect of our health.

In the last decade, science has worked to elucidate the benefits of autophagy, glymphatic filtration, and detoxification, which predominantly occur during sleep. In August 2012, the research of Maiken Nedergaard and Jeffrey Iliff and their team at University of Rochester Medical Center published their findings regarding a newly discovered system in the brain they deemed the "Glymphatic System" — more than a decade after I finished medical school.

Their report discussed how the glymphatic system in the brain was analogous to the lymphatic system of the body, in that it clears or flushes the brain of the accumulated toxins and other waste products that occur during the day, such as those which may put one at risk for neurodegenerative conditions.[97] The beta-amyloid and tau protein tangles that build up in Alzheimer's disease, and other pathological neurodegenerative conditions, are two examples of protein debris and other toxins that can be flushed out of the brain by this glymphatic system while we sleep.[95] Interestingly, this cellular housekeeping system, if you will, only seems to function to any significant degree while sleeping.

Now we know one of the reasons we need sleep! This important daily toxin removal almost exclusively happens while we sleep! Wouldn't it be cool if we had an analogous system that happened in our homes that cleaned quietly while we slept? One that did the dishes, laundry, cleaned the bathrooms, and mopped the floors? Wishful thinking, I guess.

Knowing that sleep is of critical importance, what happens if we don't get our recommended 8 hours of sleep every night?

Here is a brief list of some short-term consequences:

- Decreased memory performance and cognition
- Emotional distress (the crankiness my wife noted in me)
- Mood disorders
- Decreased quality of life
- Increased stress[*]

Longer-term consequences of poor sleep include:

- Increased risk of heart disease
- Type 2 diabetes
- Insulin resistance
- High blood pressure
- Obesity
- Dyslipidemia
- Metabolic syndrome
- Several cancers
- Even premature death[98]

It is interesting to note that shift work, such as that of a physician — or anyone who works the late night or overnight shift — is classified by the World Health Organization (WHO) as a possible carcinogen (cancer-causing). Recent reviews of such literature published in the prestigious medical journal *Lancet Oncology*, in July 2019, concluded that there is "evidence that night shift work contributes to breast, prostate, and colorectal cancer."[99]

Findings in this study were based on the work of 27 scientists from around the world in 16 different countries, who reviewed the data on this topic and found that the trend of increasing cancer risk in shift workers was from the impact of the circadian rhythm disruption, and its untoward effects on diminishing immune response, as well as increases in metabolic derangement and inflammation.[99] We will soon discuss the power and impact of optimizing circadian biology.

Now, these findings do not mean you have to change your job if you fall into this category, as I do. But you should pay careful attention to how you can stack the deck in your favor, by optimizing your circadian rhythm. I certainly took a second look at this in my life, and am very glad I did! Directly understanding circadian rhythm is essential to improving our health, because in order to optimize it we must coordinate our behaviors to match the circadian clock our bodies have been following for millennia.

When our circadian rhythm is out of whack, not only can we more easily gain weight and become more prone to chronic disease, this may even cause an early death. This got my attention about a decade ago, and I am impassioned to now share what I've learned with you.

Circadian rhythm is our 24-hour daily physiological rhythm — our biological clock. It comes from the Latin root words *circa (about)* and *diem (day)*. Interestingly, this daily rhythm is shared with many other organisms, including plants, other animals, and even the microscopic organisms that make up our gut flora and microbiota.

The primary trigger that sets off this cycle is exposure to light. This is why humans typically have a diurnal or daytime cycle. In other words, we have historically been actively performing our business during the day, and sleeping/resting from our daily activities during the night.

That is, until the light bulb screwed things up about 150 years ago. Artificial light provided the opportunity for shift work and other circadian rhythm disruptions, such as screen time, the twenty-four-hour drive-thru, and convenience stores making light, food, and jobs available around the clock. Although a very fascinating topic and worthy of an entire book, I will summarize the salient points briefly as they pertain to our metabolism and overall health, and what we CAN do about it.

Let's talk about light first, as it is one of the key factors in setting our circadian rhythm. There is an area in the hypothalamus of the human brain called the suprachiasmatic nucleus (SCN), which is the body's master clock that receives input from the eyes via the retinal nerves, specifically the intrinsically photosensitive retinal ganglion cells (ipRGCs). These special cells detect the presence of visible light, notably the blue spectrum of visible light, and can help set circadian rhythm even in those who are blind.

After these cells detect primarily blue spectrum light (at the 400–500 nanometer [nm] range) they send a signal to the SCN of the hypothalamus in the brain, which in turn signals the pineal gland to either release melatonin (when it gets dark) or stop releasing melatonin if the cells sense blue spectrum light.

According to the brilliant researcher Dr. Satchin Panda, optimizing our circadian rhythm involves two key factors. In their research within the last decade at the Salk Institute, Dr. Panda and his team have determined that exposure to light and food likely play the biggest roles in setting and maintaining our optimal circadian rhythm.[100]

Fortunately for us, BOTH factors are amenable to optimization, and we can intervene! Not only are we able to optimize our exposure to light and synchronize it to natural cues, but we can also choose to follow a similar schedule with our meals, in order to keep them both in sync with our circadian rhythm. In other words, eating during the day, and abstaining from it during the night is ideal.

In order to accomplish this, Dr. Panda recommends we incorporate some form of intermittent fasting (time-restricted feeding) into our routine.[100] I won't delve into much detail, as I've already devoted an entire chapter of this book to discussing this important health tool. But to summarize this recommendation, we must begin to mirror the daily routine of our ancestors, eating 8–12 hours during the day and fasting for the remaining 12–16 hours.

In my experience, the technique I've found most simple and effective is what I like to call a simple circadian fast, consisting of a prolonged overnight fast. This simply means not eating after dinner until breakfast, waiting 2–3 hours after dinner before bedtime (avoid eating late dinners), then waiting at least 1 hour upon awakening to eat your first meal. This mimics what our ancestors may have done before the advent of refrigeration and convenience stores. In order to easily incorporate this circadian fast, we can establish what I sometimes call a "food curfew." In other words we need to stop eating several hours before bedtime, preferably three or more to get the best results.

Dr. Panda has looked at this extensively in mice, and now in humans, and what he discovered is that incorporating some version of fasting into our lifestyle can help decrease inflammation, improve cognition and mental sharpness, decrease metabolic dysfunction and insulin resistance, and even improve chronic diseases such as heart disease and cancer. Its practice has also been linked to longevity.[100] What I've found is that one of the simplest ways to do this is with circadian fasting.

Now let us return our focus to the critically important issue of improving our sleep. I have already suggested some short and long-term consequences that occur from decreased sleep, but now I want to share the huge health benefits of optimizing it. These range from improving our daily function through increased energy, alertness, memory and focus, and quality of life, all the way to more long-term benefits, such as decreasing one's chance of suffering from metabolic disease such as insulin resistance, type 2 diabetes, high blood pressure, heart disease, and even cancer.

A groundbreaking study in September 2019 shared how improved sleep can decrease our risk of heart disease. The *Journal of the American College of Cardiology* reported that less than 6 hours of sleep a night *increases* your risk of heart attack by 20%, whereas simply extending your sleep time (if getting less than 6 hours) by just one hour *decreases* your risk by 20%.[101]

Optimizing sleep (getting your 7–8 hours of zzzz's) not only helps fight against heart disease, however. What other benefits can you enjoy? Well, you can also lose weight!

"Did you say I can lose weight just by sleeping?"

Absolutely!

Can you imagine anything easier or more straightforward than this?! In fact, in the *Canadian Medical Association Journal,* it was reported that in a six-month weight loss program, participants who slept more than 7 hours a night had 33% more success with weight loss.[102] Conversely, poor sleep (getting less than 7 hours) promotes weight gain through multiple hormonal mechanisms: increased ghrelin levels (the hormone that makes you hungry), decreased leptin (the hormone of satiety), increased insulin, and insulin resistance.[103]

Now it is coming together. It's science! Sleep affects our hormones, which consequently affect our metabolism. When you sleep less, your ghrelin goes up, and you get hungry! For example, I notice that when I work the night shift on reduced sleep I often have the "munchies." The satiety hormone leptin, which normally signals "STOP eating" to our brain, decreases and loses its signaling power when our bodies are deprived of sleep. Wonder why when you stay up late working, or binge-watching your favorite television series, you have a snack indulgence? It is because your brain is not receiving the normal stop signal from leptin, and instead getting the extra hunger or craving signal from ghrelin. Recent studies have even shown that our cravings also change when we are sleep deprived, making us more susceptible to that hyper-palatable, highly processed junk food.[104, 105]

Further interruptions include increased insulin, which then triggers insulin resistance if sleep deprivation continues. As reported by Buxton and colleagues in the journal *Diabetes*, in as little as one week of reduced sleep (5 hours a night) insulin resistance and deranged blood sugars had already ensued.[106] I even noticed this quite readily myself when I was working late nights in the hospital.

Chronically sleep deprived by regularly working the late night shift at the hospital, I experienced low energy, a decrease in my focus and mood, and I began to suffer from generalized aches and pains (a tell-tale sign of inflammation associated with insulin resistance), *and* elevated fasting glucose! Although I had not gained weight (yet) or felt typically unhealthy, I clearly noticed the beginnings of insulin resistance. It was not that I was getting older or "falling apart," but the simple fact that I was suffering from the consequences of insulin resistance secondary to poor sleep!

Weight gain has also been tied to growth hormone reduction, elevated cortisol, and other metabolic and hormonal disturbances. These are all effects of decreased sleep.[107] So, when you are not sleeping well and you get the late-night munchies, you are *not* demonstrating a lack of willpower. You are instead experiencing the powerful hormonal consequences of sleep deprivation. The salient point is: we *need* our beauty sleep, at least 7–8 hours of it!

So how can we optimize our sleep? Here are some techniques I've collected from both my study and personal and shared experience over the past decades:

- Optimal sleep begins with our daytime habits! Yes, what we do during the day affects how we sleep at night, beginning with daylight exposure. Light is everything, so exposing ourselves to natural light during the daytime and less of it at night has proven to be very helpful. In fact, only a couple of minutes of natural light exposure in the first couple of hours of the day may be the most powerful in this respect![108]

Who knew that getting a great night's sleep begins with what you do in the morning?!

- I try to minimize nighttime exposure to blue light, especially on screens, for 1–2 hours prior to bed. During the day I also try to get outside at least once, preferably in the morning, to have the sunlight hit my skin and my eyes (without wearing sunglasses) and during the brightest hours of the day (opening up the shades/windows is also helpful, though not as much). Plus, being outside gives you an added dose of what I like to refer to as *vitamin N* (if you remember, for *nature*), as well as vitamin D, which both have tremendous positive benefits.

- My bedroom at night resembles a cave like that of our ancestors, minimizing as much light as possible from entering the room when it's time to "hit the hay." This means using blackout shades and turning off all screens (computer, television, all devices that may beep, flash, or vibrate), while getting rid of night lights, LED screens of stereos, alarm clocks, or other electronics in the bedroom also helps. The darker the room the better, to optimize sleep. And while traveling, I unplug everything I can and use black electric tape to cover any extraneous light sources. I've also swapped out regular night lights in the bathroom for red lights, as they are less likely to jack your circadian rhythm.

Also remember that caves usually remain cool and have a constant temperature, regardless of the season. Our sleeping "cave" should be similar, with a room temperature somewhere between 60–72 degrees Fahrenheit, (shoot for 65) or whatever level is comfortable for you (for me this depends on how cool my wife will let me set the thermostat, as she sleeps cold already, while I tend to sleep warm).

The warmer the climate (especially in the summer months) the more difficult it is to get a good night's sleep, especially in the absence of a temperature-controlled environment. One 2019 study reported in the *International Journal of Environmental Research and Public Health* showed that high-temperature weather decreased sleep quality, causing both decreased sleep duration and shallow sleep.[109] I have definitely experienced this in Hawaii in the summer, as without air conditioning it can be difficult to get to those ideal 60–72 degrees, which has certainly affected the quality of my sleep. What has helped me then is to shower before bed and keep the fans going throughout the night.

Rounding out the cave comparison, for those who have visited a cave you'll know that they are generally quiet, so yours should be too.

- Try to limit extraneous noises. If you struggle with outside noises like the roosters crowing outside my bedroom in Hawaii or your partner snoring, try using quality earplugs to help with this. As they say, "silence is golden," and concerning sleep, I couldn't agree more.

Environment and consistency matter. Think of your sleep room as a cave, and try to keep it dark, cool, quiet, and as free from distractions as possible! These sleep habits are important for overall sleep hygiene. The two most significant circadian rhythm disruptors are blue light and eating just before sleep time. So, to repeat, begin with minimizing blue light exposure 1–2 hours before sleeping, and try not to eat within 2–3 hours of bedtime. Just as you should have a blue light or *screen curfew*, you should also have a *food curfew*! This will make a big difference, and is an easily implementable tool that is both simple *and* free!

- Avoiding significant amounts of liquid intake for 1–2 hours before bed also helps limit bathroom awakenings. In addition, although alcohol may aid in *getting* you to sleep, it decreases the *quality* of sleep, especially if drunk within two hours of bedtime, so generally try to avoid its use.

- Drinking caffeine earlier in the day instead of the evening is best. Enjoying caffeine within six hours leading up to bedtime (sorry after dinner coffee drinkers) decreases both the quality and duration of sleep.[110]

- If you *must* have a little something before bed, try to keep it to a no-calorie beverage, such as a small cup of water, herbal tea, or decaf coffee. Keeping your drink low in calories will help your body get into fat-burning mode sooner, as well as helping you have a more restful sleep, as you won't be in full digestive processing mode — digestion is notorious for disrupting sleep. (Remember the food curfew?)

- I have also found that regular exercise during the day improves the quality of sleep. Try to avoid doing so within 60–90 minutes of sleep, though. If I do need to fit in my exercise in the evening, I try to keep it to a moderate intensity level or I just do a simple walk. This recommendation is consistent with a large 2019 meta-analysis reported in the *Journal of Sports Medicine*, which determined that evening exercise is okay at a moderate level, and is best concluded at least sixty minutes prior to bedtime.[111]

- If you are sleep deprived from work-related experiences and are in need of a daytime nap, try to limit it to a "power nap" of 30–60 minutes. Napping longer during the day has been shown to decrease sleep quality at night.

The first priority should always be to strive for the requisite 7–8 hours a night. Limit napping unless you are sleep deprived is a great goal too. Getting 7–8 hours of continuous sleep at night is always better than sleeping less in the evening and trying to make up for it during the day.

Always listen to your body, and practice mindful sleeping practices you find beneficial to your particular situation. This supersedes textbook teaching. The most important human being is YOU, so always listen to your body.

Remember that whatever routine helps you attain a relaxed state before bed is the one for you. It will take experimenting, planning and a little tweaking, but your routine should certainly be individualized. Do what works for you!

- I have found that incorporating an ease down routine to prepare for a restful sleep is key. Some people enjoy an evening bath, a relaxing routine of meditation, reading a physical book (preferably not on a screen), journaling or other quiet time practice before bed. All of these techniques are beneficial. Personally, writing in a gratitude journal is a great wind-down ritual for me. Given that we are putting away the screens 1–2 hours before bed, and not eating for at least 2-3 hours, we should have plenty of time for any wind-down ritual(s) of choice.

If you still struggle with sleep after having incorporated all of the above into your routine, some natural foods and supplements taken within two hours before bed may help. Camomile tea, magnesium, ginkgo, glycine, valerian root, L-theanine, lavender, and melatonin are great options. If you do use any of these, always try to use the smallest recommended dose, for the shortest duration possible. I have known many people to take excessive melatonin, for example, and experience untoward effects such as daytime drowsiness, dizziness, nausea, and headaches. I personally find melatonin quite helpful when used to help with jet lag and use it as needed.

- A technique I've recently found beneficial in reaching a mindful sleep experience is the practice of earthing or grounding (walking outside barefoot). What's great about it is its simplicity. Just slip out of your shoes and go for a barefoot walk in the grass, sand, or sidewalk. Or simply stand outside on the earth for a few minutes. I try to practice this almost daily (though find it occasionally difficult in the winter if I am in the snowy mountains), and it has been very helpful to my overall well-being, mood, and sleep. This simple technique of earthing, or grounding, has also helped me significantly minimize jet lag, by adjusting my circadian rhythm while traveling and crossing time zones.

This ancient practice has been shown to improve sleep, normalize circadian rhythm, promote the shift to the restful parasympathetic nervous system from the stressed of fight and flight, decrease pain, increase heart rate variability (what many sleep devices monitor), speed up wound healing, and improve blood circulation by decreasing blood viscosity, as reported in the *Journal of Inflammation Research* in 2015.[112] Who knew this simple, free technique of slipping off your shoes and grounding could have such a plethora of benefits?

Remember, optimizing the light/dark circadian cycle creates space for restful, rejuvenative sleep. The benefit of having an ease-down ritual before sleep is just as important as what we ingest before we lay our heads on the pillow. Returning to our ancient lifestyle roots by optimizing the two largest and most important regulators of circadian biology, our exposure to light and food, and the timing thereof, are fortunately under OUR control! We cannot simply wait to *"sleep when we are dead."* Because ultimately, achieving optimal health *while* we live should be our goal, yes?

Now that we have outlined an action plan for restful sleep that contributes to our overall health and long-term weight loss, let us move on to exercising our muscles, our body, and our heart.

Shall we dance?

CHAPTER 6

The Magic of Movement

> *"Walking is man's best medicine."*
> - **Hippocrates**

Who's up for a natural, safe, and simple physiologic high? I mean a full-on endorphin rush and natural, endogenous cannabinoid high? Exercise (movement) can be that simple and rapid game changer to positively affect your mood, state of health, and emotional well-being. It can reverse your low energy and downtrodden spirits, bouncing you into an energized, pumped-up stratosphere in no time. Optimal physiology is critical and I can't think of a better way to enhance it than to move!

Our mental and emotional state are everything, and I have not found a more quick and powerful way to change my realtime state than getting in some physical movement and heavy breathing.

Surfing; running; intervals; weight lifting; biking; hiking; climbing; tennis; skiing; snowboarding; resistance training; push-ups; pull-ups, and taking a walk, have all been great for setting my body in motion. Each of these simple activities lends great strength to the powerful locomotion of your overall health. Come on, do I really need to say what trainers, doctors, health coaches, and nutritionists have been telling you for years? YES, the *secret potion is constant motion* that will help you accomplish long-term health and weight loss as well.

Have you ever experienced a down day? You know the kind, when nothing seems to go right, leaving you feeling bummed, or "down in the dumps"? While experiencing this, you might have decided to go outside for some fresh air, take a walk, run, bike ride, or do a quick workout of some kind. How did you then feel? All of a sudden your state improved, and you felt so much better, right? Truly like a whole new person. Yet this is not a coincidence, this is science!

In fact, this happened to me even while writing this book. I literally had the entire first draft completed, and because of a fluke in the saving and transferring process, the whole manuscript was lost! The WHOLE THING. Shocked, mortified, and angry, my emotional state was at rock bottom. And what did I do? I went surfing!

This immediately changed my state. I emerged from the waters reinvigorated, refocused, and able to approach the dilemma with clarity. I wish I could say I recovered that manuscript. Nope. But my quick change in mood from a surf session, and remaining active through repeated movement and exercise, helped me continue optimizing my state as I rewrote the manuscript.

I do not think there is any way I could have otherwise empowered myself to do this, if I did not have the power of movement to keep my spirits high, help me maintain resolve, and keep my commitment grounded. Indeed, managing your state is everything. You can change your physiology and present state in as little time as it takes to do a quick bout of exercise or a movement routine. The natural feel-good hormones and neurotransmitters working in tandem with the brain, supercharging *BDNF* release (brain-derived neurotrophic factor), are the real deal. THEY LITERALLY SAVED THIS BOOK!

In fact, an interesting study reported in the journal *Psychoneuroendocrinology* reported on the stress-buffering effect of acute exercise. In this intriguing study, they took two groups of young people (one group that had just exercised for 30 minutes and one group that had not) and exposed them to two stressful scenarios: a scary image, and a difficult mental math problem. The researchers studied their responses by recording the levels of the stress hormone cortisol, as well as functional MRI imaging, to document the young people's brains' responses to the stressors.[113]

As if it was not enough to have them do the difficult math problem in their head, they also exposed them to those scary images while doing the math! Sounds cruel to me. What they found was that the group that had exercised for thirty minutes right before these stimuli had lower levels of the stress hormone cortisol in their blood, as well as diminished stress responses in their brains.[113] The exercise they had just completed significantly buffered the stressful events![113, 114]

Have you had a similar experience? No, not looking at scary images while doing a mental math problem! Maybe you have had a stressful event in which your mood was then positively changed with a bout of exercise or movement? Often when I find myself getting a little testy, I do a quick review of my day. Did I fit in some time for movement? Did I complete my favorite exercise routine? Frequently, I have not. Yet I find that as soon as I do I am literally a new person. Just ask my wife or my kids for that matter. It's not just kids who need to get their "wiggles out," if you know what I mean!

Exercise or movement can be very successful in elevating mood — in both the short term and as an adjunct activity for treating anxiety, depression, and other mood disorders. It can also aid in drug addiction recovery, acutely improve cognitive performance, and decrease the risk of cognitive decline demonstrated in Alzheimer's disease.[115] This brain-enhancing effect is a result of the neurotrophic factor *BDNF*. It's like a miracle drug for the brain, natural and powerful. Its release during exercise promotes brain growth and plasticity, which results in quicker learning, enhanced memory, and a decreased risk of developing neurodegenerative diseases.[116]

We can truly be healthier and expose ourselves to less risk of acquiring a chronic disease, and potentially live longer, if we exercise regularly. Ruegsegger and Booth delineated at least forty chronic health conditions that exercise improves, in their article entitled "Health Benefits of Exercise."[116] See the table below:

This is a list of forty conditions caused or worsened by the lack of physical activity, with growth, maturation, and aging throughout life span. All forty conditions *improve* and/or decrease in incidence with regular physical activity.

1. Accelerated biological aging/premature death	21. Hypertension
2. Aerobic (cardiorespiratory) fitness (VO2max)	22. Immunity
3. Arterial dyslipidemia	23. Insulin resistance
4. Balance	24. Large arteries lose more compliance with aging
5. Bone fracture/falls	25. Metabolic syndrome
6. Breast cancer	26. Nonalcoholic fatty liver disease
7. Cognitive dysfunction	27. Obesity
8. Colon cancer	28. Osteoarthritis
9. Congestive heart failure	29. Osteoporosis
10. Constipation	30. Ovarian cancer
11. Coronary (ischemic) heart disease	31. Pain
12. Deep vein thrombosis	32. Peripheral artery disease
13. Depression and anxiety	33. Preeclampsia

14. Diverticulitis	34. Polycystic ovary syndrome
15. Endometrial cancer	35. Prediabetes
16. Endothelial dysfunction	36. Rheumatoid arthritis
17. Erectile dysfunction	37. Sarcopenia
18. Gallbladder diseases	38. Stroke
19. Gestational diabetes	39. Tendons being less stiff
20. Hemostasis	40. Type 2 diabetes

I would venture to say that the overwhelming majority of us will have one or more of the above conditions, and they *all* can benefit from this free and simple strategy — movement!

Exercise is amazing, and I highly recommend it. My favorite benefits out of the many available are the spark of clarity it lends to my mental health, a reduction in stress, and an overall uplift to my everyday well-being. The increase in energy I feel after a bout of exercise is a natural high I love to enjoy. The musculoskeletal strengthening and growth from mindful movement and exercise also helps prevent sarcopenia, improves relaxation and sleep, and increases libido and sexual function in both women and men![117, 118]

My personal goal with exercise is to make movement a part of my daily routine a minimum of five to six days a week. I simply feel and sleep better when I get some movement every day, and I often do a light walk on days six and seven too. You may be asking, "What type of exercise is best?" My knee-jerk response to this is, "The one that you will do!" Choose an exercise or activity you enjoy participating in. This will ensure you will do it the longest. The longer you commit to an exercise routine, the healthier you will become for your future best self. And the longer you will be able to keep doing it by staying active! My personal goal is to be the first human to *still* be surfing at 100 years old!

Many benefits from exercise can be enjoyed with even a moderate level of activity. Once you have committed to doing 5–6 days of exercise a week, you can experiment with an activity that works best for you, in order to experience enjoyment and accomplish the exercise goals you have set.

Don't just choose an activity because you *think* it is the best exercise to help you lose weight. Pick something that you can picture yourself doing on a regular basis. Whichever activity you choose in the beginning, be daring and remember to change it up sometimes. Variety in your movement routine is the spice that'll keep you actively strong and desiring more!

Recent studies have shown there are additional benefits to mixing up your exercise routine. Resistance training in particular (any version of weightlifting, using resistance bands, or body weight resistance exercise) has been shown to improve metabolism and increase metabolic rate, reduce fat and improve lipid levels, and improve physical performance and cognitive abilities. It also improves numerous metabolic parameters, such as decreased hemoglobin A1C, insulin resistance, and visceral fat (the bad intraperitoneal belly fat that puts us at risk for heart disease, diabetes, and other chronic health conditions).[119]

But don't overdo it! Have you heard the saying, "too much of a good thing can be a bad thing"? Well, this can be easily applied to exercise. What I am getting at is this: extreme levels of exercise can elevate your cortisol (the stress hormone) to an excessive amount, which can be this "bad thing." Excessive cortisol as a result of overtraining is metabolically disadvantageous, as it raises glucose and insulin, both of which increase the risk of insulin resistance if those levels remain high too often.

Remember, overall exercise is a good thing! But it is not effective if your diet and eating habits remain poor. Exercise alone will not often accomplish weight loss. If your diet remains unchanged, and exercise is employed as your only weight loss tool, many people will find they actually gain weight. Dietary change is a much more effective weight loss strategy, with time-restricted feeding and exercise most effective when complimenting this. Again, contrary to popular belief, you CANNOT exercise your way out of a CRAPPY diet!

Say for instance you have just run for twenty minutes, and then did five minutes of lunges. This is approximately equivalent to 150–200 Calories burned, depending on how hard you run and how intense you do your lunges. But then, you decide to have Oreos® for dessert after lunch to reward yourself (there are about 150 Calories in two Oreos®) — you just exercised, and you feel extra hungry, so it's okay right?

Yet with this cookie indulgence, you completely negated your exercise potential for weight loss. If you ate more than 3 cookies (come on, you know you ate half the pack), you may wind up with a net *gain* of Calories, not to mention inflammation and feeling less than awesome afterwards! An increase in hunger after exercise is normal, but try not to indulge in empty calorie rewards, as this can be counterproductive to your weight loss goal.

One of my favorite stories which elucidates this principle occurred to a friend of mine, well-known fitness trainer and lifetime health advocate Vinnie Tortorich, a couple of decades ago. He recalls, during his university studies in health sciences and kinesiology, monitoring a young and fit individual perform a VO2 max fitness experiment while on a treadmill, running all out and uphill. After nearly 20 minutes of near-maximum effort, they calculated he burned approximately 230 calories.

Shortly after this experiment, Vinnie found himself eating lunch and sharing a small bag (1.69 ounces) of M & M's® chocolate candies with a fellow student. He remembers reading the label, which showed that the small bag of candy was 230 Calories — the same burned in that maximal effort bout of exercise, where this well trained athlete appeared to be suffering, was extremely winded, and ultimately threw up. It dawned on him at that very moment that exercise, in most cases, is a near impossible solitary mechanism for weight loss, if dietary habits are unchanged.

One of the early chapters of this book highlights the important principle of "Food First," when related to weight loss and overall health, because this really is where the magic begins.

> *No amount of exercise can*
> *compensate for a crappy diet.*
> *NONE!*
> *Never has, never will.*

(Read that again.)

Begin your journey by improving the QUALITY and TIMING of your food. Once you are comfortable with your new schedule and menu, incorporate optimal sleep and exercise for their additional health benefits.

For now, however, take a deep breath, and congratulate yourself for embarking on an exercise regime — that's AWESOME! And now that you know to focus first on what is at the end of your fork, exercise should be a fun enhancement to your weight loss goals.

Did I say fun? Absolutely! Exercise, if it is to be done daily, is much more successful if you enjoy doing it. I enjoy many outdoor activities, from hiking to tennis, but when I can't do any of these, I simply go for a walk! I love walking! Not only is it a great form of movement for your whole body, but you can easily change pace with intervals, lunges, burpees, or whatever you desire. And, it is *free*, requires *no* gym membership, and can be done almost *anywhere* in the world!

Remember, variety is KEY. Just like our mind, spirit, and palate often crave some variety, so does our body! So, MIX IT UP! Overuse of certain muscle groups, joints, and tendons can occur from excessive single sport activities (think monotonous repetitive running for "x" amount of miles or minutes on the treadmill, and never changing the routine, slope, or length of the run). Besides, why would we want to miss out on so many benefits from other sports and activities?

Doing something every day is also key. My general recommendation is to exercise six days a week, but on the seventh day, you can do a light after-dinner walk — no formal workout.

The simple movement of walking reminds me of two different trips my wife and I took to Italy. Even though there seemed to be a Pizzeria or Panaderia on every corner, no one seemed overweight or obese! We also noticed that people walked almost everywhere. After dinner is when we would see most Italians — taking a walk! They may or may not have realized that this simple postprandial (after a meal) walk not only helps with digestion but improves insulin sensitivity and decreases that feared spike in glucose and insulin that can lead to low energy, brain fog and more cravings. This simple practice of walking after meals is one of the most powerful I have encountered and I strive to incorporate it into my personal and family's routine as often as possible, ideally, multiple times a day!

This simple activity of walking has been shown to have a positive, continuous linear mortality benefit, as reported in 2015 in *Journal of Epidemiology*. They studied adult males from 65 to 74 years, with or without a major critical disease (heart disease, cerebrovascular disease, and cancer), and found that all groups with adverse medical history experienced a significant mortality benefit related to daily walking. They concluded that adding a walk to a daily routine may improve longevity and successful aging.[120] Simple, and universally effective, walking is a high value, low entry form of movement.

Beyond a decreased risk of heart disease and the inherent mortality benefits, most impressive to the positives of walking are the short and long-term benefits to your brain health. Indeed, walking can also decrease your chances of acquiring a neurodegenerative disease such as Alzheimer's and other dementias. Our brains may shrink with age, but remember that it can be treated like a muscle. Our brain *does not* have to decrease in size just because we get older. So just keep moving!

A fascinating truth is that the very areas of our brain (the prefrontal cortex and hippocampus) that shrink most with age — on average 1–2% per year after age 55 — are the MOST likely to respond to exercise or movement! Moreover, these are also the areas that are most commonly affected by Alzheimer's and other dementias.[121] So, if you want to keep your senses and your druthers, get out and move. And do it daily!

Going back to what daily activities optimize the use of our bodies, I am a firm believer in exercise or movement with attention to the functional aspects. What I mean here is picking activities that help in creating and preserving function. Dumbbells for biceps curls, bench presses, or doing the same paced run or monotonous gym session five days a week may work for the beach body but likely will not cut it for lasting health and preserving our functional needs.

When I think of activities that promote function, I think back hundreds or thousands of years, and consider what we as ancient humans did. We ran, we walked, we sprinted in short spurts, we lifted heavy things, and carried them to build shelter, bent over to pick berries or tubers, climbed trees, and fished. More recently we tilled and cultivated with our backs, legs, arms, and hands. We used our whole bodies to live and work.

One of the best ways we can incorporate functional movement into our daily activity is by using resistance training (RT). It excites me to learn that the scientific community is finally beginning to see the benefits of resistance training, rather than solo daily cardio as I was taught during medical training. A review published in 2019 in the international journal, *Health Promotion Perspectives,* found when specifically looking at individuals fifty and over, that resistance training improved mental health, decreased body aches and pains, and improved emotional, social, and physical roles in life functions.[122] They recommended working on all major muscle groups two or more days a week, which helps with maintaining muscle mass and bone density. Even if you are not over fifty, resistance training carries the same solid benefits for your body. Resistance training for the win!

Exercise is the part of the day I look forward to most. I know I will feel amazing afterward — sharp, focused, mentally ready to tackle anything, and juiced up for the win. If your exercise is leaving you feeling overly tired or super hungry, you may need to adjust your approach.

Focus on preparation, with a good, solid diet that is focused on whole foods with adequate protein, healthy fats, and low to moderate carbs. Initially try to maintain carbohydrate consumption between 100–150 grams a day, then you can adjust as needed. (Remember, a dependency on excessive carbohydrates can leave you hungry shortly after meals or snacks, and can potentially stall your metabolism.)

If you are feeling famished at the end of your workout, you are either exercising too hard or you may still be heavily dependent on carbs, and your body has not quite kicked into the fat-burning mode. You can easily change this by decreasing your carb intake a notch, and monitoring your workout with a heart rate monitor to make sure you do not exceed your maximum heart rate. I've also started to eat protein prior to my heavier work out sessions and noticed I feel stronger and perform better.

A maximum heart rate is calculated by the simple formula: **220 minus your age in years.** You should shoot for close to this number though not exceed it during your higher-intensity cardio or resistance exercises. Don't try to go much beyond your number, as this can become more "stressful" to your body, thus elevating cortisol, glucose, and insulin. This may terminate your fat burn potential, as well as increase your chances of damaging your metabolism from this stress, and its associated insulin resistance, if you consistently overdo it.

Speaking of stress, we are about to take a deep dive into it.

So, who's ready?

CHAPTER 7

Stress to Challenge

> *"It's not stress that kills us, it's our reaction to it."*
> **–Hans Selye**

Let's start with some good news about stress! *We* get to decide if it will be a positive challenge and growth experience, or a detrimental slump, a principle that is both beautiful and empowering. We are the *only* ones who can attach meaning to whatever stress we may feel or experience. We are in charge of the outcome. We've got this!

A landmark study demonstrating this principle was published in the journal *Health Psychology* in 2012. Here Keller and colleagues reported that it was not so much the presence or absence of stress that affected people adversely, but their BELIEF or perception about the stress, that to a great extent determined the outcome.[123] Let me explain: almost 80% of those included in the study (147,897) experienced measurable (mild, moderate, severe) stress at some point during the year, and 38,087 (about 20%) reported almost none.

Those who had the most stress, AND believed the stress they experienced was bad for their health, increased their risk of premature death by 43%.[123] Based upon their belief alone. And those who also had the highest level of stress and did

NOT believe that stress was bad for them, not only did NOT have increased mortality, but this stress proved positive and protective for them! Keller and colleagues went on to determine that during the study period (nine years) the number of deaths attributed to this negative belief was about 20,231 per year. Thus, the *meaning* we attach to our stress is extremely significant.

Stress is one of the major factors of life that plays a significant role in our everyday health. I believe most of us are either experiencing some level of stress right now, or will experience stress in the next 12 months. The real concern is HOW we respond to it. That is the key to how it may affect our health and our life!

The negative physical effects of stress include a greater susceptibility to illness; lack of energy; interruptions in sleep; headaches; poor judgment; weight gain or weight loss; depression; anxiety, and more. It is now time to address this battle, and take meaningful action to ensure our experience is a positive one that lends viability to our long-term health. In order to relieve stress, we need to know what is causing it, as well as what factors are dictating the impact. Then, we need to create solutions that will alleviate these factors.

There are several ways one can respond to a stressful situation or stimulus. There is the classic *fight or flight* sympathetic nervous system response (the view of the stress as a threat and all the correlated positive and negative hormonal surges that follow); the *freeze and paralyze* response (deer in headlights reaction); the *challenge* or *growth* response (the view of stress as a challenge or game to be won or conquered, overcome or accomplished), and *the tend and befriend* response (think Bob Marley "every little thing gonna be alright"). One can either respond to stress positively or negatively. Remember, WE get to decide!

Positivity and happiness are a choice! I truly believe that *life happens for you, not to you.* The power of positivity is real, not only in the moment, but can literally increase your lifespan. A review published in the journal *Social Science Medicine,* in November of 2015, concluded that being happy helped you live longer. Those who classified themselves as "not happy" increased their chances of dying by 21%.[124] Indeed, happy people live longer.

In addition to happiness, having a positive future outlook, a network of social support, and trust in relationships with others also appears to give one protection from the stressors in life. Returning once more to the *British Medical Journal,* Rosengren and colleagues studied the effects of having positive support while dealing with stress in 1,016 men aged 50.[125]

They found those who experienced stressful events preceding the survey — difficulty with a family member, loss of a job, financial trouble, having to move homes, or being involved in a lawsuit — all increased odds of premature death *only* in the group that lacked a good social support network. In the group with a high amount of social support, there was no evidence of a mortality effect on those who experienced one or more of the listed stressful events. Clearly, then, having emotional support is protective.[125]

People who are happier, and live day by day with a positive outlook on life, live longer. Having stressors, but good emotional support to deal with them, serves as a protective barrier against an increased risk of mortality.

So, what is going on here? How can we explain this? Well, let's take a moment to briefly look at the physiology of stress.

The classic categorical stress response that triggers the sympathetic nervous system response (fight or flight) causes a surge in cortisol, affecting glucose and insulin levels, which directly affect metabolism, causing inflammation in the short-term. With increased inflammatory markers like interleukins and TNF-alpha, stress also has negative long-term effects on the brain — causing shrinkage (atrophy also with decreased BDNF levels) and decreased connections (reductions in synapses), especially in memory areas such as the hippocampus and amygdala.[126] Stress can also suppress the immune system, predisposing you to increased risk of infections and cancer.[126]

Becoming physically sick after a highly stressful event in your life is not an uncommon reaction. Heart attacks, damage to the gastrointestinal (GI) system (causing leaky gut), endocrine abnormalities such as adrenal fatigue, chronic fatigue, and a decrease in growth hormone and thyroid levels are all cases I have witnessed as a physician, with stress being a root cause.

Now that we know some negative effects of stress, how do we approach it with a challenge or growth response, rather than the typical stress response? Well, this depends on how we view it, or what meaning we attach to it. Let me give you a personal example. When I was in medical school I had weekly exams on Monday mornings — what a terrible way to consistently ruin my weekend, right? Not exactly.

Instead, I chose to view this as an opportunity to prepare for a game I wanted to win. And studying for the exams became the warm-up exercise I knew would help me do this. I began visualizing the end — acing the test, and how awesome that would feel. I used this energizing emotion of accomplishment to help propel me forward during studying, and carried that positive affirmation with me while taking the exam. Results? Drumroll, please…

I regularly aced my exams, and graduated at the top of my class. Now, I do not use this example to brag, but instead to demonstrate how I learned to turn a stressor into a positive challenge. By looking at the future with a positive mindset (viewing the potentially stressful exam as a mere challenge or game I wanted to excel at or ace) as I prepared for and took my exams, I reversed a potentially negative outcome. This is a similar approach I imagine that elite athletes take as they prepare for the big game or event they excel in, both with the positive mindset and future visualization as well as viewing it as a challenge that they *can win*.

Findings from a study into this very preparatory approach to exams were reported in the journal *Advances in Medical Education and Practice* in 2019. The researchers studied two groups of students from a Public Health Master's program. In one group they offered additional sessions on both mental and practical skills, to help reduce the anxiety of exam taking, while the control group just had the normal class sessions. What they found was that the intervention group, the one that had the extra sessions, not only experienced less anxiety related to test taking, but also performed better as a result.[127]

What I have found in life is that if we plan ahead and practice how we might respond to stress even before it happens, leaning on our inner growth response, we will likely produce a positive outcome.

Like many, I also used to be afraid of public speaking. Yet everything changed when I decided to adjust my approach, and view it as a growth or challenge experience — something that could be exciting and exhilarating. With this mindset, I rehearsed repeatedly, and found this changed my nerves tremendously before I gave a talk or speech in front of an audience. Once again, a challenge-response is an energizing and growth approach to stress.

Now, physiologically, what makes the difference between the traditional fight or flight response, and a challenge or positive growth response to stress? Recent scientific data suggests that the hormone oxytocin, the so-called "cuddle" hormone, plays a significant role. It is so potent and multi-faceted that it can easily be regarded as an anti-stress hormone.

Oxytocin is released when triggered by labor, breastfeeding, sex, stroking, warm temperatures, positive social interaction, positive thinking, and even eating.[128] It is believed that oxytocin induces well-being by stimulating a dopamine release in the nucleus accumbens of the brain, as well as decreasing the stress response in the amygdala and hypothalamic-pituitary-adrenal axis (HPA).[128]

An oxytocin release produced during the growth or challenge response can actually protect us from the adverse effects of stress mediated by cortisol and adrenaline. Oxytocin can also help us to become more resilient (like in the case of the study referred to previously with those who had social support upon experiencing significant life stressors), and it can encourage us to seek social connections to help us cope during times of significant stress. This oxytocin release is powerful and has been a game changer in my experience. I truly believe it is what can miraculously mitigate the adverse effects of stress, *if* we seek to encourage its release through our social connection, positive outlook and emotional resilience.

In fact, I often like to refer to this powerful tool of connection as another version of vitamin C, the C being for *connection*. In fact, in my studies of the *Blue Zones* (where the longest lived peoples reside) the most powerful shared element and factor in their longevity, in my opinion, is this same power of *connection*. I have been to both Costa Rica and Italy where there is an increased percentage of centenarians residing. In addition, what I have personally witnessed there is the strong sense of community, family and connection that the people have and it is very much alive, well and palpable. People are not just people, they are your friends, loved ones, aunts, uncles, relatives, neighbors, and *all* have a place in the community and are connected to one another in some way or in many ways. It is a beautiful thing to experience and one that we would do well to emulate.

Don't worry, there won't be a quiz on all the physiology and biochemistry, though I include it to help paint the picture of the many positive and far-reaching effects of oxytocin on stress. It can alter an event from one that is stressful and draining, into an energizing, positive growth, and resilience scenario. Once again, the good news is *we get to decide* how to deal with stress and what meaning we attach to it!

Next time you feel stressed or overwhelmed, step back, take a deep breath, reassess, and imagine how you can incorporate a positive mindset and outlook to frame the stress. Remember, life does not happen *to you*, but *for you*. I challenge you to take inventory of events that trigger you, and those that bring you joy and peace. Make sure to create more space for the latter!

I have personally found that disconnecting from technology and taking a walk in nature; doing breathing exercises, mindfulness and meditation, or yoga; writing in a gratitude journal, chatting with a friend or family member, and participating in exhilarating locomotion activities — surfing, mountain biking, skiing, playing a good game of tennis or ping pong, or even just sitting quietly as I catch a sunrise or sunset with those I love — seems to do the trick. Connecting with both nature and people I care about has been a game changer in my life and has earned this an honorary vitamin C in my book, for *Connection*!

So, take a moment and make a list of the things that bring you joy, peace, and positive vibes, and commit to doing more of them! Let the positive vibes of oxytocin flow!

Now, let's look at the final powerful practice that will help optimize our health, and prevent disease, by caring for our gut.

CHAPTER 8

Change Your Gut, Change Your Life

> *"All health begins in the gut."*
> — Thomas Hemingway, MD

Your gut bacterial makeup needs a balance of diverse colonies of healthful strains of good bacteria, and less bad bacteria. Less of the *Firmicutes*, more of the *Bacteroidetes*, for example. This balance reduces cravings for unhealthy foods, and the neurohumoral bacterial sabotage, that alters your mood when the less healthy bacteria send chemical messages to your brain, making you crave that hyperpalatable junk food. Once again, it is not a lack of willpower, but proven science of the gut.

Beyond the roles in immune function, digestion, metabolism, and vitamin and nutrient production, the role of the gut microbiota in brain health (and endocrine and cardiovascular health) are also beginning to be understood. Nearly every physiological function has an important interaction with our gut health. The root of the presence or absence of disease can often be found in our output, so let's get into how we can optimize our gut health.

To do so, we don't have to get dirty, at least not yet. If we fail to take advantage of these tools to promote our gut health, and we succumb to SIBO (small intestinal bacterial overgrowth) and dysbiosis, there is always the extreme option of eating poop from a healthy individual (fecal transplant). Though I think most of us can agree we wouldn't want matters to become so drastic!

Instead, I have some top gut health tips for you to follow, so let's go!

Why You Should Care About Your Poop

> *The presence or absence of disease can often be traced to our poop, literally!*

When Hippocrates said nearly 2500 years ago that "All disease begins in the gut," he may not have been too far off. Considering that what we eat affects almost every aspect of our health, and that the foods we consume have intimate contact with the gut (by passing directly through it), this statement makes complete sense. In addition, tremendous connections are rapidly being discovered regarding the role of our gut microbiome. Specifically, our gut bacteria and other flora which make up our collective microbiota directly impact a number of diseases, versus healthier states of our bodies.

So, why should one care about these microscopic bacteria, fungi, protozoa, and viruses that only make up a couple of pounds in our intestinal tract and our daily excrement? For one, we are clearly outnumbered! Yes, they outnumber us both in the numbers of cells and in the amount of genetic material they contain. For example, it has recently been estimated that there are in the neighborhood of 38 trillion bacterial, viral, and fungal cells that live in or on our body, and about 30 trillion human cells.[129]

It was previously estimated that these non-human cells (bacterial, viral, and fungal) outnumbered us by up to 1000 to one. More recently, they seem to be on par with the number of human cells that make up the human body. In either case, we are as much bacteria, viruses, and fungi as we are human cells. Considering that we are only half human by the number of cells, greatly outnumbered in terms of genes (there are at least 150 times more genes in our foreign microbiome — bacteria, fungi, and viruses — than human genes[129]), and inundated with foreign matter, we should probably pay attention to these organisms that make up our microbiome, wouldn't you think?

Besides the fact that we are clearly outnumbered by genetic material and the number of foreign cells that make up our respective microbiome and microbiota, recent scientific data suggests that these microscopic organisms play a significant role in our health. For example, chronic diseases such as the inflammatory bowel-related Crohn's disease and ulcerative colitis, as well as type 2 diabetes, insulin resistance, heart disease (cardiovascular disease), and colorectal cancer, have all shown connections to the gut microbiome.[130]

Not surprisingly, the microbiome (the combined makeup and genome of these microorganisms) is largely dependent on environmental, *not* genetic, factors. For instance, identical twins do not necessarily have the same microbiome, despite having an identical human genome. In other words, it matters more what environmental factors and behaviors are at play, such as what we eat and how we interact with our environment, than what genes and microbiome we inherit.[131]

We are in control of these factors. Therefore, we are in control of our microbiome, and the resulting disease or health that ensues, to a significant extent. This empowering notion excites me, as we are not bound by this microbiome. We can instead decide, by our habits and behaviors, what its makeup contains. Though we cannot change our inherited human genome, we CAN change this acquired microbiome through the actions we take. Health, or disease, truly does begin in the gut!

Let me give you an example. Rothschild et al., in their article in the highly respected scientific journal *Nature*, titled "Environment Dominates Over Host Genetics in Shaping Human Gut Microbiota," showed that the phenotypes — observed characteristics of body size (body mass index [BMI], waist-to-hip ratio, fasting glucose levels, glycemic status, and cholesterol levels such as high-density lipoprotein [HDL]) — are significantly correlated to one's microbiome.[131]

That is to say, they discovered that the makeup of the gut microbiome in those studied was a major determinant of their weight, blood sugar status (metabolic health), and cholesterol levels. This proved that our individual microbiome is largely dependent upon *our* choices of what we eat, and what we do or don't do.

WE GET TO DECIDE!

Take the case of a detailed twin study performed in the U.S., again reported in the prestigious journal *Nature*, where it was found that the diversity of the gut microbiome correlated well with obesity or lean status, rather than simply with the genetic predisposition of being twins. They found across all the twins studied (over 150), either monozygotic or dizygotic, as they tended towards being overweight or obese, that their respective microbiome became less diverse. Conversely, the lean twins (even in the pairs where one twin was lean and the other overweight or obese), tended to have a more diverse microbiota.[132] Once again, diversity matters, especially in the gut!

Furthermore, when their human microbiome was given to naive mice (via fecal transplant), they adopted the phenotype of the twin of origin, despite being fed the exact same diet, both in calories and macronutrient makeup. In other words, when mice were given the stool transplant of the lean twin, they became lean, and when they got the stool from the obese twin, they became obese, despite the fact that both groups had the exact same number of calories and the same diet![133]

You want your gut microbiota, and the genes expressed there (the microbiome), to be as diverse as possible! Diversity is best achieved by an appropriate amount and mix of natural real foods in your diet working in tandem with healthy behaviors.

A 2019 study reported in the *British Journal of Nutrition* also concluded a similar trend in body weight, as related to the diversity of the microbiome. The researchers evaluated the diversity of the gut microbiome in college students, and found it to be inversely correlated with weight gain. As weight increased and trended towards obesity levels in these college students, the amount of diversity in the gut bacteria decreased. The converse showed lean students had more diversity in their gut microbiome. Diversity truly is the spice of life for our microbiome![134]

The health of our gut indeed matters, just as Hippocrates proposed 2500 years ago. So how do we attain greater diversity — more good bacteria phylum (*Bacteroidetes*) and less of the other (*Firmicutes*)? It all starts at the end of your fork:

What you feed, will breed.

In other words, the groups of bacteria you prefer to feed will grow and spread throughout your gut, ultimately affecting your entire body through the downstream effects of gut health. Without delving too deep into the weeds of how every food type affects the gut microbiota (and they all likely do in some way), let me share with you some common threads that will give you the tools to make great choices when creating your new "menu." Remember, the goal is to healthily feed yourself, and by extension your gut microbiota.

Let's go!

Your Gut Bacteria May Be
Sabotaging Your Waistline

A diet high in processed foods (especially refined and processed carbohydrates and industrial seed oils), most commonly consumed in a Western or standard American diet (SAD), generally leads to decreased gut health (less diversity in the microbiome), more *phylum Firmicutes*, and less *Bacteroidetes*.

It is estimated that the standard Western diet comprises approximately 60% highly processed foods.[135] Sadly, this number is reported to be even higher in children and adolescents, where up to 67% of their diet is from highly processed foods.[136] These numbers should frighten you, yet simultaneously, let them instill in you the courage to *not* be part of this SAD statistic!

Not only does a highly processed, carbohydrate-rich diet lead to less diversity in the gut, but also a greater probability of increased intestinal permeability, or "leaky gut." A "leaky gut" leads to increased inflammation in, as the name suggests, the gut, *and* the body, by boosting endotoxemia and its associated inflammation (due to bacteria and their associated toxins crossing the gaps in the lining of the gut, and into the bloodstream, through leaky junctions caused by poor dietary choices).

This can contribute to a myriad of chronic diseases: obesity, type 2 diabetes, heart disease, and cancer. The SAD or

Western diet consists of many processed foods which also contain additives and sweeteners. These unhealthy foods are often manufactured using processed fats (seed oils and hydrogenated oils) — the fats that have been shown to lead to an unhealthy bacterial ratio (dysbiosis), leaky gut, and chronic inflammation, that contribute to a myriad of chronic diseases.

In a 2018 article for the journal *Nutrients*, Zinocker and colleagues discussed this newly discovered phenomenon at length.[137] They argued that the processed nature of the Western diet (standard American diet) is highly involved in an increased incidence of obesity and metabolic disease. The highly processed characteristic of the Western diet, in addition to the large number of additives (i.e., processed oils, artificial colors, flavors, emulsifiers, and sweeteners), has shown to be extremely pro-inflammatory, while playing a major role in altering the composition of the gut microbiota; leading to the dreaded condition of dysbiosis.

Interestingly, the gut bacteria favored by these highly processed foods (dense in calories, though nutrient-poor) likely also contribute to both weight gain and dysbiosis. They literally sabotage the signaling that occurs between the gut and brain.

Let me explain: remember the less favorable bacteria, like *Firmicutes*? They care only about their survival, so they send signals to the brain, encouraging carbohydrate and processed food cravings, in order to promote their own survival and longevity, not caring about the resulting propensity towards inflammation, dysbiosis, and metabolic disease. Remember it's simply for their survival though we suffer from the collateral damage.

A landmark scientific report in the journal *Bioessays* details specifically how gut bacteria, in order to promote their own survival, manipulate our cravings through neurochemical signaling. *Firmicutes* have been shown to do this by several fascinating mechanisms. They are able to produce chemical messengers that generate our cravings for certain foods, to either promote their growth and fitness, or suppress the craving of healthier foods that grow their competitors, like the more healthful bacteria *Akkermansia*.

Firmicutes have also been shown to cause dysphoria, to the point we finally give in to eating the foods they want us to. Don't follow the theme — they want to multiply! And if they multiply, they win. Your journey to gut health continues to be compromised if you eat processed foods that increase the presence of these harmful bacteria.

The junk food craving we have is not necessarily our own. Gut bacteria are capable of literally hijacking the vagus nerve (the main gut-brain neurological connection) to promote their own survival, at the expense of our diminished health.[138] These bad gut bacteria are capable of manipulating the reward and satiety pathways, thus making us crave unhealthy foods. They also produce toxins that can alter our mood, and can even promote changes in our taste receptors.

> *No, it is not that we are weak and lack*
> *willpower or self-control — it's science!*
> *Yet another way we can be manipulated*
> *by the physiology of our gut bacteria,*
> *unless we do something about it.*

Let's talk about artificial sweeteners, shall we? Splenda (sucralose) is a favored sweetener in the U.S. You yourself may enjoy it in your coffee, tea, or your go-to iced drink? Well, it has been shown to adversely affect the gut microbiome, and lead to increased inflammation. In fact, all of the studies I reviewed for the writing of this book demonstrated some degree of negative effects of artificial sweeteners on the microbiota.

In the scientific journal *Frontiers in Physiology*, Bian and colleagues looked at acceptable intake levels of sucralose. They found that the compound not only increased tissue inflammation, and elevated pro-inflammatory gene expression, but it also led to significant liver inflammation or hepatitis.[139]

Saccharin (Sweet'N Low) presented similar behavior for the gut microbiota. It has been linked to gut dysbiosis, and a decrease in the beneficial bacteria *Akkermansia muciniphila*.[140] Remember, *Akkermansia muciniphila* is a very beneficial strain of gut bacteria, known to help with weight loss and leanness, improved mood, decreased inflammatory diseases, as well as decreasing insulin resistance. It is definitely a gut bacteria you want! Yet artificial sweeteners interrupt the presence and performance of these good bacteria.

Recently, *Akkermansia muciniphila* was studied in relation to obesity, and was discovered to be directly linked to weight loss, improvement of insulin sensitivity (decreasing insulin resistance), increased metabolism, and decreased inflammation.[140] It also helps preserve the mucosal barrier, or lining of the gut (thinner than the width of a human hair), to help prevent increased intestinal permeability ('leaky gut'). A few corresponding problems that may arise from a compromised mucosal barrier are inflammation, autoimmune and immunologic diseases such as food allergies, and increased susceptibility to infection.

Yet the perils of the Western diet and its dependence on artificial ingredients do not stop there. Other studies looked at aspartame (Nutrasweet) and its negative effect on our gut microbiota. A May 2021 study, reported in the *International Journal of Molecular Sciences,* discussed artificial sweeteners and their effect on the gut microbiota. Researchers found that all three sweeteners (saccharin, aspartame, and sucralose) had negative impacts on gut health.[142]

There were direct pathogenic (harmful) effects on two common gut bacteria: *Escherichia coli* and *Enterococcus faecalis.* The sweeteners showed an increase in biofilm (making them less susceptible to antibiotics and more virulent), and an increase in adhesion and production of cytotoxins, which kill host cells.142 These artificial sweeteners, though "generally regarded as safe (GRAS)" still wreck our microbiota at levels that make us increasingly susceptible to infection and microbial invasion, leading to liver and systemic inflammation setting up for a myriad of issues. I want no part of this — do you?

Next time you want that artificially sweetened zero or low-calorie bubbly beverage, or prefer to add your favorite sweetener to your hot refreshment, take a moment to contemplate the effects it will have on your gut! It certainly gives me pause.

So, that was artificial sweeteners. Now, how about another common additive — emulsifiers? Food emulsifiers also have the potential to harm our gut flora or microbiota, as well. In another study outlined in *Nature*, it was reported that relatively low concentrations of two commonly used emulsifiers — carboxymethylcellulose and polysorbate-80 — cause inflammation, and play a role in obesity and metabolic syndrome. It also increased the risk of contracting significant colitis (inflammation of the colon lining).143

The researchers attributed these findings to the emulsifiers' harmful effect of decreasing microbial diversity, thinning the protective mucus layer of the gut lining (leading to 'leaky gut'), and increasing bacterial adherence (making them stick more easily to the intestinal cells in order to invade them), that leaves the gut in a generalized pro-inflammatory state with increased lipopolysaccharides (LPS or endotoxin).143

Endotoxin, or LPS, is known to contribute to inflammation, leaky gut, and several chronic inflammatory conditions: obesity, type 2 diabetes, non-alcoholic fatty liver disease, and cardiovascular disease.[143] In fact, most experts would recommend a diet that does not significantly elevate endotoxin or LPS levels, to avert these dangerous and potentially deadly inflammatory conditions. This recommendation is an anti-inflammatory natural whole foods diet: no processed foods or artificial additives (sweeteners, colors, flavors, and emulsifiers).

Given the findings of so many adverse effects that artificial additives have on our microbiome[144] — dysbiosis (altered proportion of gut bacteria, leading to unhealthful bacteria outnumbering the good bacteria), intestinal hyperpermeability (leaky gut), and increased inflammation of both the gut and the body — I definitely recommend caution in their consumption.

How about eliminating them from your diet altogether? Well, I was not able to find a single unbiased study showing any health benefit to using artificial additives. Being given "generally regarded as safe" status (GRAS) by the FDA, should not sway your decision to do all in your power to avoid them as you strive toward optimal gut health. Remember many harmful substances over the years have been initially given GRAS status such as the hydrogenated oils, though they have later proven to be severely detrimental and toxic to our health. Why take the risk?

The quality of our food trumps everything. For the health of our microbiota and ours, let's start reading our food labels! I know for me, this research has justified my new habit of reading the ingredient list before I decide to buy. Additives have become so increasingly common in foods many of us eat regularly. Now, more than ever, it's critical to read the labels when purchasing food. Paying special attention to the ingredients list is paramount because the labeling and marketing can be severely misleading and flat out deceitful. I have noticed dozens of times that many "healthy" dressings or sauces, for example, will state they contain olive oil and thus are health promoting when if you take a moment and read the ingredients list you will find that olive oil is much farther down the ingredients list than the more prevalent, and more toxic vegetable seed oils.

Make good choices for you and your gut. Remember, *we* are largely in control of the makeup of our gut bacteria and the resulting microbiome. It all depends on how *we* care for and feed it. Remember, *what you feed will breed,* for better or worse. Likewise, *we get to decide* what environment exists in our gut by the things *we* eat, *our* physical habits and behaviors, and *our* exposure to environmental helps or hindrances. Additionally, we will soon discuss powerful strategies to optimize this gut milieu.

The Power of a Healthy Gut Microbiome

Let's take a step back to appreciate the magnitude of the gut health issue, and how it can be optimized to enhance not only the health of our microbiota, but indeed, ours as well. Let's take a moment to appreciate the extent and magnitude of this critical system. What makes up our gut, and just how big is it anyway?

Take, for example, the case of a friend of mine, whom we will call Jane, who came to me asking for help with her constant cravings for sweets, poor sleep, brain fog and trouble concentrating, lack of energy, inflamed and painful joints, and mood challenges with both bouts of anxiety and even depression.

I began by asking her about her diet and behaviors. What I found was that her diet, not unlike many Westerners, was predominantly composed of processed or prepared packaged foods coming from a bag, box, or with a barcode. She also had poor sleep hygiene, and her exercise routine was not regular. These are all factors that predispose one to dysbiosis, or an imbalanced gut microbiota favoring those not-so-healthful strains like the *Firmicutes*.

We worked on changing her diet, initially with a type of elimination diet, then began incorporating lots of real, whole, and unprocessed foods, especially with increased fiber content as well as adding probiotic-rich foods like kimchi, kefir, and tempeh. We also applied the techniques explained already in this book, regarding sleep and circadian rhythm optimization and regular movement, and within a few months her dysbiosis had resolved. What's more, nearly all of her symptoms explained above completely disappeared, along with significant improvements in her mood and mental health — *without* any prescription medication!

Paying attention to our gut health or microbiota is so critical, for a myriad of reasons. Aside from the sheer volume of cells and genes associated with our gut microbiota and microbiome, the surface area of our gut can pose a significant help or threat to our health, depending on how we care for it. The tremendous surface area that our gastrointestinal tract encompasses is literally an exposed open route to the outside world, by virtue of anything we put into our mouths, healthful or toxic.

Our gastrointestinal tract, from mouth to anus, is approximately 30 feet in length, and the surface area is anywhere from the size of a studio apartment to that of a tennis court, depending on what source you read. In either case, it is a significantly large surface, indeed, our largest organ, where the outside world comes into contact with our internal world, and literally exists only one cell away from our circulatory system or bloodstream.

The extensive surface area of the gastrointestinal tract is made up of many rugae (folds in the stomach and intestinal lining). In addition, even smaller, finger-like projections called villi on its inner surface allow for an expansive interior surface area, perhaps as much as 200 square meters, if it were entirely stretched out. Therefore, the gastrointestinal tract amounts to the largest surface area in the human body. And by sheer size, volume and proximity, it becomes the most susceptible to invaders, and toxins.

Our gut is also available to process and receive stimuli from the outside world, through the foods we eat. Therefore, it is definitely a double-edged sword, in that it can either be exposed to healthful foods and nutrients and aid in their digestion and metabolism, or be exposed to unhealthy foods, toxins, and pathogenic invaders. And whether the former or latter transpires is largely OUR CHOICE!

Keep in mind that the lining of this tennis court-sized entity is very, very thin — only one cell thick (much thinner than a human hair). This single-cell layer is critical in facilitating the absorption of nutrients. If healthy, it is tight enough to prevent potential pathogens (harmful and disease-causing invaders) from permeating or penetrating this thin and susceptible barrier.145

When our gut functions properly, and the intestinal border (tight junctions) remains intact, it is able to properly metabolize and absorb nutrients, while keeping the potentially harmful bacteria and allergens out. Yet when it becomes increasingly permeable, as in the case of leaky gut, (increased intestinal permeability) the potential for bacterial invaders and allergens crossing the border increases, and disease-promoting inflammation becomes problematic. A modern example in many people would be gluten. Endotoxin from the bacteria or allergens could cross this narrow gap between intestinal cells, made "leaky" by gluten, causing havoc on intolerant gut systems.

In order to maintain optimal gut health and the intestinal border's integrity, we must pay attention to what we eat and drink, as this directly correlates to our gut health. If we do so, we will not only have protection from potential invaders and allergens, but also benefit from the myriad of digestive and metabolic functions that optimal bacterial diversity can afford us. We will dive into this further in a moment, to discuss the foods and practices that will promote optimal gut health.

Now that we know the magnitude and powerful influence of the microbiota, our microbiome, and the absorptive surface of the gut, what are some of the functions a healthy gut microbiota provides us? The variety of functions are wide, and only recently becoming more elucidated, appreciated, and shared. When I was in medical school, the main focus with respect to gut bacterial health was on keeping the pathogenic (harmful) bacterial species at bay, as they could potentially become dominant after a course of antibiotics, for example. Such as occurs with the well known problem of C. *difficile* colitis. We now appreciate there are many more important functions and interplays within a healthy gut flora, in relation to the rest of the body, than simple retardation of pathogens.

One of my favorite examples of a newly discovered and very exciting feature of our gut bacteria is the notion of the gut being our "second brain." Gut bacteria are responsible for a range of signaling processes along the connections between our gut and our brain. These are often referred to as the gut-brain axis, or the gastrointestinal enteric nervous system — commonly referred to as our "second brain." What is not often appreciated by physicians and others in the health profession is that ninety-five percent of the serotonin in the body is in the intestinal tract, and its modulation and signaling processes are affected significantly by the gut microbiota.

Let's revisit those helpful gut bacteria *Akkermansia muciniphila*. Their interplay with the neuroendocrine system has been shown to affect serotonin production, released from enterochromaffin cells of the gastrointestinal tract that affect the corresponding signals occurring between the gut and brain. A recent study reported in the peer-reviewed journal *Scientific Reports* noted that *Akkermansia muciniphila* was found to modulate genes that regulate serotonin production and expression in the colon and hippocampus of the brain.[141]

The researchers found that when mice were given this bacteria, it promoted increased serotonin concentration in the gut, as well as enhancing signaling throughout the gut-brain axis. They concluded that this technique of optimizing the presence of *Akkermansia* in the gut should be considered as a useful tool in therapeutic strategies to help with serotonin-related disorders: mood disorders like anxiety and depression; gastrointestinal disorders such as inflammatory bowel disease, including Crohn's, and ulcerative colitis.[141]

Indeed, numerous studies have looked at the connections between bacterial diversity in the gut and the presence or absence of mood disorders. Generally speaking, it has been found that a decreased bacterial diversity in the gut microbiota is correlated to an increased prevalence of anxiety and depression.

In a recent review by Huang et al. in the scientific journal *Frontiers in Genetics*, researchers discussed the important bidirectional interaction between gut bacteria, our microbiota, and the brain via the gut-brain-axis, as well as neuroimmune and neuroendocrine pathways.[146] This interaction plays a key role in the signaling between these microbes and the brain, through neurotransmitters like serotonin, dopamine, and choline. Our serotonin, dopamine, and choline levels are important parts of brain health and the challenges that develop in the form of mood disorders. Through their extensive review, the researchers discovered that certain bacterial species tended to be either more or less present, depending on certain conditions, and that both diversity and short chain fatty acid production were generally reduced in the gut bacteria of those suffering from brain health challenges (anxiety, depression, bipolar).

In other words, those suffering from brain health challenges like depression tended to have decreased bacteria diversity in the gut, and decreased levels of healthful bacteria that produce short-chain fatty acids (SCFAs), which feed intestinal cells. People in this category also tended to have more pro-inflammatory gut bacterial genera, and less of other healthful bacteria such as *Lactobacillus, Akkermansia,* and *Bifidobacterium.*

This is super exciting! Not only does it reinforce the tremendous role healthy gut microbiota play in our overall health, but it provides a potential pathway for natural non-pharmacological treatment approaches to brain health challenges — depression, anxiety, bipolar, and other related mood disorders. No offense towards pharmaceutical solutions (they can be life-saving in the right context). But their efficacy in brain health challenges, in my experience as a physician, leaves a lot to be desired with respect to efficacy and side effects.

Knowing there may be other treatments available, such as using a food as medicine approach (paying close attention to gut health), incorporating exercise and movement, optimizing one's sleep, and practicing stress modification, could be the most powerful therapeutic approach yet! This approach is just beginning to be understood and appreciated, and the future is bright!

> *Not only do our gut bacteria help in this magnificent "second brain" gut-brain axis communication, but they also produce many necessary vitamins and nutrients vital to food digestion, metabolism, and assimilation.*

For example, gut bacteria can produce many B vitamins like thiamine (B1); riboflavin (B2); niacin (B3 or nicotinic acid); pantothenic acid (B5); pyridoxine (B6); biotin (B7); folate (B9), and cobalamin (B12).

B vitamins must be regularly consumed, or produced in our gut, as we have no significant appreciable storage form for them in the body. Therefore, it is very important to seek sources in our diet, such as avocado, asparagus, spinach, lentils, mushrooms, fish, as well as grass-fed and well-raised chicken and beef, including organ meats, which are all excellent dietary sources of B vitamins. Our healthy gut microbiota can also produce the very important Vitamin K — critical for coagulation hemostasis (appropriate blood clotting) in the body.

Gut bacteria also help digest many of the nutrients we consume into more bioactive and available forms, such as with the plant polyphenols, and are also involved in fueling the intestinal cells with those critical short chain fatty acids (SCFAs). These SCFAs are produced from the fiber we eat, to make acetate, propionate, and butyrate, which have been shown to positively promote better intestinal and microbiota health which leads to less "leaky gut."[147]

In this same vein, certain bacteria can even produce natural folate (vitamin B9) when certain strains of lactic acid bacteria (LAB) like *Lactobacillus delbrueckii,* or the *Bifidobacterium* like *B. longum,* are added to milk to produce yogurt. This fascinating study was performed by researchers on Argentinean yogurt, in which the lactic acid bacteria, *Lactobacillus delbrueckii,* produced natural folate (not folic acid).[148]

Besides being the natural and much more bioavailable form of folate (methylated folate) — formed from a real food source instead of a supplement — the yogurt also contains a folate-binding protein, which further improves folate bioavailability.[149] This is a huge benefit. There is ongoing research in efforts to produce a natural folate-rich yogurt made by this helpful bacteria.[150]

This essential vitamin production by our gut microbiota plays a key role in the digestion and metabolism of proteins, bile acids, and plant polyphenols (antioxidants).[151,152] Polyphenols have been an exciting topic within recent studies, as they have been shown to offer protection against certain cancers, cardiovascular disease, diabetes, neurodegenerative diseases, and osteoporosis. Interestingly, without the contribution of the gut microbiota, many of these benefits may go unnoticed to some extent. This is because the human body cannot adequately digest polyphenols on its own, without help from the gut bacteria.[152]

Polyphenols are present in fruits, vegetables, dark chocolate, herbs, spices, and wine. Perhaps the most well-known and popularized of these polyphenols is that of *resveratrol*, the potent polyphenol in grapes and berries, which can be found in red wine. An upside of your favorite bottle of red!

This potent antioxidant (of the stilbene class), popularized by longevity expert Dr. David Sinclair, has been proved to have amazing benefits, due to its significant anti-inflammatory properties. Moderate consumption of resveratrol (from red wine, grapes or berries) benefits our heart and brain. There is also evidence that it supports positive anti-carcinogenic and anti-aging effects. If you are not a wine drinker, no worries, as you can also get resveratrol from grapes and various berries.[206] Another reason to finish your meal with a handful of juicy colorful berries!

Another potent polyphenol antioxidant is one that comes from the cacao bean: dark chocolate. Its antioxidants act as an anti-inflammatory. Many positive benefits include a decrease in heart disease, lower blood pressure (it improves blood flow), a decrease in insulin resistance, and improvement of lipid metabolism and brain function.[153]

Antioxidants in cacao improve blood flow through the release of nitric oxide (NO) — the same nitric oxide that erectile dysfunction treatments are targeting.[154] Improvement in blood flow benefits the entire body. From the cardiovascular system to cerebral blood flow, these antioxidants demonstrate positive effects on our heart and brain health.

Benefits of cerebral health include benefits with the neurodegenerative diseases Alzheimer's and Parkinson's, likely derived from the combination of anti-inflammatory effects, improved blood flow, and increases in the brain-derived neurotrophic factor (BDNF) hormone.[154] Chocolate for the win!

Having amazing anti-inflammatory and antioxidant effects, is it any wonder these polyphenols in cacao positively benefit the microbiota in our gut?! To expand, they increase the presence of helpful strains of bacteria in the gut that lead to decreased inflammation throughout the body. A study by Andujar and colleagues reported significant improvements in colitis (inflammation of the colon lining) from cacao administration. They felt that it was likely due to cacao's effect on decreasing the inflammatory cytokines responsible for the inflammation in colitis.[155]

Having listed the positive effects of cacao on our heart and brain, I would be remiss not to mention that polyphenols have also been proposed as an aid for managing obesity by several distinct mechanisms. Firstly, cacao can decrease the hunger hormone ghrelin. In addition, it interacts with the hormone adiponectin in our fat to help protect us from insulin resistance. When we consume dark chocolate, for instance, its polyphenol protein modulates the adiponectin hormone, which decreases fat synthesis and enhances fat metabolism.[156,157]

In other words, properly sourced and real cacao (in dark chocolate and high-quality cocoa) can be super beneficial — to weight management and gut health! Now, I am certainly not suggesting that we start going crazy with traditional chocolatey treats here, but if we stick to well-sourced, high-percentage dark chocolate (over 70% cacao) — read the label! — by eating a small amount (between 10–20 grams a day — one or two squares of a bar) we can maximize the benefits of delectable dark chocolate, without contributing to our waistline. One of my favorite sweet treats is a handful of sea salt macadamia nuts chased by one square of dark chocolate. Truly divine!

Again, these powerful antioxidants come from real foods. So isn't it great they also happen to be some of the most enjoyable on the planet? Red wine, berries, and chocolate — wow! Who knew I'd be recommending incorporating these important powerful phytonutrients: the polyphenols? If you stick to real foods, you'll be surprised how much your body, mind and your gut will benefit.

There are so many tasty real foods available on this amazing planet. A lot of these plant-based polyphenols, like many other nutrients, have also been synthesized for mass production and sold in supplement form such as resveratrol. But, why not try them from their whole food source? Not only may this certainly be more enjoyable, but likely more bioavailable, beneficial and affordable as well. Remember, FOOD FIRST, and then supplement to fill in the gaps.

> *There is nothing that can replace*
> *a high-quality, well-sourced, REAL FOOD diet.*
> *NOTHING.*

In addition to their nutrient-producing and metabolizing effects, the gut microbiota and microbiome are also intimately involved with our immune system function, as their balance and diversity have been directly related to our health. It is generally accepted that the majority, 70-80 percent, of our immune system resides in our gut. Here, the immune cells constantly interact with the gut microbiota, which presents both neural and hormonal signals through the multitude of messengers they produce.[207]

It is often said that what is present in the gut, through diversity of bacteria and foods, is what provides the majority of the training for our immune cells. Hence, the more diverse your diet and microbiota, the better trained your immune cells will be to not only better resist infection but also to stay strong and resist much of the allergy and auto-immunity issues that are becoming more commonplace today.

Gut bacteria produce the all-important SCFAs (short chain fatty acids) from the fiber we eat. These are the ever-so-important acetate, propionate, and butyrate (the top three most prevalent SCFAs), which serve many vital functions for our immune health. These SCFAs not only serve as an amazing food source for our intestinal cells, but they also modulate immune cell function, like the helper T cells for example, and can also decrease inflammation.

These SCFAs can also stimulate the goblet cells in the intestinal lining to secrete the protective *mucin*, in order to maintain the integrity of the very thin intestinal border through this mucin activity, while maintaining the tight junction integrity. Based on interactions with pathogens, allergens, and other substances, the microbiota are also extensively involved with the signaling that activates the immune system.

Through diverse pathways, our microbiota is involved with both innate and cell-mediated immunity.[151] Again, the role of the microbiota and microbiome is intricate and far-reaching, making it truly essential to the health of the host — us!

The Original Superfood for Gut Health: Fermented Foods!

Talking about optimizing the health of our gut microbiota, it truly may be the most amazing resource and partner in our overall health. And using a gardening analogy of *seed-weed-feed* can help us to understand the significance of our gut health. If we were growing a garden in our backyard, we would take simple steps to ensure the survival of our plants, vegetables, herbs, and fruits. We would select the best seeds, we would position them in the best mulch — making sure the soil is nutrient-rich — and we would rid them of weeds and other invaders that may harm their growth.

In our "gut garden," we need to take similar care of the microbiota that exist for our overall health. Paying careful attention to how we *seed, feed, and weed* our "gut garden" creates space for a positive impact on our daily health and vitality, as well as our ability to avoid and fight disease and illness. Now, in order to influence the bacterial makeup of our gut and its diversity, we need to first seed it with the best helpful bacteria available, which can be obtained both from the foods we eat and with probiotic supplements to fill in the gaps. So, let us explore seeding our gut garden (our microbiota).

We begin by eating the most healthful varieties of beneficial microbes. We should strive to eat 1–2 servings of fermented foods daily: yogurt; kefir; some cheeses (like aged cheddar, feta, goat cheese and gouda); sauerkraut; kimchi; tempeh; natto; pickles; kombucha; buttermilk, and organic sourdough bread from a starter. Fermented foods can not only add to the healthy gut flora as a probiotic, hosting bacteria such as *Bifidobacterium* and *Lactobacillus*, but fermentation also helps us by making nutrients in the parent foods more bioavailable during the pre-digestion stage. Moreover, it increases the activity of certain nutrients, such as the previously discussed polyphenol antioxidants.[158]

Remember what I said about red wine? Rich in polyphenols, right? Bacteria fermented with polyphenolic compounds become more bioavailable and active (they are converted into more active metabolites), and therefore more usable for us! Fermentation can also reduce toxins and anti-nutrients, in such foods as natto, tempeh, and miso, which are soy-based. In their fermentation process, the phytic acid found in soy and its products — which can act as an anti-nutrient by impairing absorption of such minerals as iron, calcium, and zinc — content is reduced, while still retaining the helpful antioxidant qualities.[159,160,161]

Additionally, the pre-digestion of the soy by the bacteria in tempeh, natto, or miso, also "supercharges" its antioxidants by metabolizing them into more active antioxidants, enabling them to better absorb the damaging free radicals and superoxides.[162] Thus, fermentation not only decreases the anti-nutrients in soy like phytic acid which can decrease the nutrient absorption of other important vitamins and minerals, but also makes the beneficial nutrients such as the anti-oxidants; much more bioavailable; a true win-win!

Now, all that means is when you eat fermented foods, like miso or tempeh, for example, the nutrient value is far higher than it would be if you consumed a whole soybean, such as edamame. This gives the antioxidants "superpowers," if you will, enabling them to effectively protect us against dangerous free-radicals and reactive oxygen species that contribute to disease and premature aging.

It is interesting that only in the last two decades have these fermented foods become hugely popular in our American diet. They have literally been used in our "human" diet for millennia, as long as 10,000 years or more. In fact, it is believed these fermented foods were likely humankind's original processed foods.

This original fermentation not only helped with the preservation of alcohol, yogurt, and meats but also enhanced food safety and organoleptic properties (gustatory activation of the senses during eating).[158] It is currently accepted that fermented food, due to its effect on pre-digestion and bacterial metabolism stages, can provide enhanced nutritional and functional properties, beyond the ingredients in its original food base. It truly makes the end-product, fermented foods, more beneficial than the starting ingredients in an exponential way where two plus two may equal twenty on a scale of nutrient density!

Besides containing helpful probiotic bacterial strains in the end product (freshly baked sourdough bread, yogurt, kefir, cheese and red wine), fermentation itself can produce even more bioavailable and nutrient-rich metabolites.[160] Some of the bioavailable antioxidants and nutrient metabolites identified in fermented foods may include those that also have blood sugar-balancing potential in addition to the powerful antioxidant benefits noted above.

A balanced blood sugar level directly affects blood pressure and energy levels. Increased anti-hypertensive (lowering of our blood pressure), anti-diabetic, and anti-allergenic properties in the final fermented food product, thus makes these foods a powerhouse of probiotic bacteria for our gut garden.[160]

The processing and bacterial digestion that occurs during microbial fermentation makes food both nutritious and also potentially less harmful to our gut. The soybean-based food examples above contain lectins, and some people experience adverse effects from lectins in soybeans and other sources. The fermentation process of soybeans contributes to making their nutrients more bioavailable, by diminishing their potential toxins as well as the lectin effects. Let's focus more for a moment on the brilliance of fermentation!

Personally, I prefer kimchi, which is made from fermented cabbage. There is just something about the spicy Korean seasoning I really enjoy, and this particular dish fully awakens my taste buds. Remember the organoleptic properties of fermented foods originally described millenia ago? I have lived in Hawaii for almost three decades, where kimchi is a staple — that likely didn't hurt. And while I discovered my children love it as well, I made another observation between kimchi and my kids. In my experience, when kids eat fermented foods from an early age, it decreases their desires and cravings for sweet foods later.

Taking steps to ensure my children had a healthy gut from a young age created space for better overall health as they developed. Through probiotic-rich foods like greek yogurt, kimchi, poi, and kefir, as well as supplements, which were all introduced into their diet as toddlers, they have not craved sweets or junk food nearly as much as their contemporaries. Keep in mind this also stands as a demonstration of how early maintenance can make a huge difference in overall gut health. (Remember, the techniques outlined in this book can serve as an action plan for you to change your health.)

This should make sense, as by doing all of this my children have populated their gut garden with good bacteria, which crowds out the bad ones which prefer processed foods and sweets, and can hijack cravings. It's science! So, if you want your kids to prefer health-promoting real whole foods, get them started young (as toddlers) on fermented foods like yogurt, kefir, poi, kimchi, and the like, and you can expect them to not crave sweets as much.

This has certainly been the case with my children, and I am reminded of it every year at Halloween, as they get so excited about dressing up and getting their treats. But since they typically don't eat many treats on a regular basis, or even crave them, a day or two later they are either forgetting about the candy or asking to just toss it, without any desire to eat their haul. I also have often found their candy a year later in their closet in a zip lock bag, well preserved, without having been touched after Halloween night!

Gustatory traditions of eating fermented foods have been a part of many cultures over the millennia. Depending on what source you reference, before the "invention" of alcohol, yogurt may have been accidentally discovered by herdsmen, transporting bags of milk in canteens made of animal stomachs on the backs of camels in hot climates. References to it go as far back as 6,000 B.C., in Ayurvedic scripts from India.[163]

These ancestors were definitely onto something when they added fermented foods to their diet. They may not have readily understood the science behind fermentation (existence of microorganisms, bacteria, yeast etc.), but this newly discovered mechanism served them well. Every culture in the world developed its own identifiable fermentation process as cultural interactions expanded, and eventually a greater understanding of the science behind it was formed. From the original, likely accidental discovery in the famed canteens made of animal intestines transporting milk by the Middle Eastern traders, to the Turkish "yoğurmak" and its purported use by Genghis Khan's Mongol army, yogurt was here to stay.[163]

Accidental discovery or not, it likely did not take long for our ancestors to realize that using fermentation was not only an excellent technique for preserving food like milk, but provided quite excellent nutritive benefits and sustenance. Those who built the Great Wall of China are said to have survived off of a diet consisting largely of sauerkraut — another fermented cabbage — and rice, thousands of years before the Germans adopted it.[164]

Today, there are thousands of fermented foods and beverages readily available for our enjoyment. It has been estimated that more than five thousand different fermented foods and beverages are consumed worldwide![165] How many fermented foods have you tried, or made? Given there are literally thousands available, here is another case of my desire for us to focus on *adding* rather than subtracting from our diet and providing delicious, tasty and nutritious foods on a daily basis! Remember food is meant to be enjoyed and savored, regularly!

An interesting review by Tamang et al., titled "Fermented Foods in a Global Age: East Meets West" in the journal *Comprehensive Reviews in Food Science and Food Safety*, itemizes many of these fermented foods by country of origin, and the list is extensive.[161] What a super interesting, detailed list this is! This long list of fermented foods from various cultures solidified the notion of the cultural and nutritional significance of these powerful superfoods over the centuries. More importantly, I was inspired to try more! My palate has only tasted a dozen or two thus far, and my checklist keeps growing! There are literally thousands of types of fermented foods to sample worldwide. Which ones will you try this week?

A great review of some of the more well-known fermented foods was published in the May 2019 issue of the scientific journal *Nutrients*. Here the authors, Melini *et al.*, reviewed the current studies and research on probiotic-rich foods: kefir, kombucha, sauerkraut, miso, natto, tempeh, soy, kimchi, sourdough — and discussed the physiology of their probiotic and nutritional benefits.[158]

These benefits include: increasing the antioxidant activity of the food (fruits, vegetables, milk, meat, and fish); lowering blood pressure; increasing available vitamin content, as well as anti-diabetic properties. I really feel like we are just beginning to scratch the surface of the benefits of this amazing, time-honored superfood!

What I also enjoy about fermented foods is that there are a multitude of them, around 5,000, across many different cultures, with a plethora of interesting and delicious flavors — each one holding a beneficial property. Remember, I still have many I need to try! There are literally thousands of them!

Another great article published in the journal *Frontiers in Microbiology* took a look at various fermented foods: cheeses, milk products, vegetables, meats, grains, and various drinks — from around the world.[166] This article serves as a great tool to remind us of not only the extreme variety of fermented foods available, but their numerous health benefits.

From making key healthful ingredients such as antioxidants and bioflavonoids more readily available to us, to decreasing anti-nutrients and toxins like lectins, they are paramount to our health.[166] I want to try even more now! Are you with me? Let us discover this culinary path together, and delight in the many amazing benefits these foods have to offer our palates and our gut. They are interesting to eat, and we can savor them together. Let's jump-start our healthy gut garden with the power of fermentation!

There are so many of them to incorporate into our diet. Taste them. Try them. Cook with them. Adding in a new one each week of your new journey towards better health will not only enhance your sensual pleasure of gustation, but positively affect your gut and your life. Add some of these powerful probiotic-rich foods to your diet today!

Here is a short list of some common fermented foods (some I have already mentioned), that should be fairly easy to obtain and incorporate into your diet: yogurt; kefir; buttermilk or another cultured milk; cheese such as aged cheddar, gouda and feta; kimchi; sauerkraut; tempeh; miso; natto; kombucha; pickles and pickled vegetables, like brine olives; kvass; apple cider vinegar, and sourdough from starter.

Remember, ADD more than you subtract, and get excited about the variety, activating your senses and reveling in the health benefits! The more diverse your palate and plate are with your new menu (real, whole, natural, and fermented foods), the more diverse your microbiome and the better your overall health! Make a list today of the ones you want to try, and gradually add to it!

As I mentioned, your gut bacterial makeup needs a balance of healthy strains, of both increased good bacteria and less of the bad ones. Less of the *Firmicutes*, more of the *Bacteroidetes*, for example. This balance reduces cravings for unhealthy foods, triggered by the chemical messengers sent by the less healthy strains of bacteria, which can sabotage your senses and alter your mood.

In the *Journal of Nutrition*, a detailed review in 2020 carefully evaluated 19 different studies, which show that the fermented foods we eat can alter the composition of our individual gut microbiota. It was suggested that regular consumption of fermented foods may represent a potential avenue to counter the pro-inflammatory effects of gut dysbiosis in both its prevention and treatment, potentially altering the composition of the gut bacteria.[167] This presents a clear connection between the foods we eat and the ultimate makeup of our gut. This was a really exciting discovery for me, and I hope it is for you too. Better living through gut health!

Seeding our gut with healthful probiotic-rich foods is just the beginning. As you begin this journey, remember your aim is for long-term benefit. After seeding the garden, one must feed it. Fermented foods and probiotic supplements supply valuable nutrients for a healthy gut garden. EAT your fermented foods, and supplement if needed. This will help grow a health-promoting gut garden to avoid bacterial overgrowth in the small intestine (SIBO), and prevent bad strains of bacteria from outnumbering the beneficial ones (dysbiosis).

Now, I briefly mention probiotic supplements, and have personally witnessed the benefits of using them from time to time. Over the years I, my family, and others I am personally connected to, have taken various forms of these supplements, and I can honestly report their worth. Now, they are not to *replace* a whole food diet, but instead, as we have discussed, to fill the gaps.

Although there are numerous studies on the benefits of specific probiotic strains in specific pathological health conditions, there is less information on the routine use of probiotics in an otherwise healthy population. One recent review article in the *European Journal of Clinical Nutrition* examined forty-five different studies on otherwise healthy subjects. It concluded that supplementing with probiotics in healthy adults can lead to transient improvement in gut microbiota concentration, while supporting the role of probiotics in improving immune system response, bowel movement and stool consistency, as well as vaginal lactobacilli concentration.[168]

This is an exciting time, as we are only just beginning to witness the numerous effects (good and bad) of the microbiome on human health. And future research and treatment for various clinical diseases and health conditions can only improve our outlook. Feeding our gut garden by providing it with good bacteria via fermented foods, and supplements if needed, is one important way to ensure its health. But make sure you continue to take care of this intestinal, health-promoting garden, by giving it more of what it needs.

What else do the good gut bacteria like to eat? Prebiotic-rich foods with fiber are their staple food of choice.

These are foods high in starch-resistant prebiotic fiber. Remember, we are feeding ourselves *and* them. Therefore, we should pay attention to our preferences as well as theirs, especially the healthful bacteria. Our cravings that may come from the less beneficial strains of bacteria are most likely found in the SAD staples of processed foods. However, helpful bacteria tend to like prebiotic fibrous vegetables. So what are those?

These are the root and fibrous containing vegetables and fruit, such as asparagus; Brussels sprouts; apples and bananas (especially green or unripe bananas); onions; garlic; leeks; greens such as kale, spinach, and chard; Jerusalem artichokes; roots such as chicory, burdock, yacon, and konjac; seaweed, and seeds such as chia, flax, pumpkin, and sunflower.

Now, you don't have to eat all of these, just pick your favorite ones and try to eat two servings each day. This is the fun part, finding which of these delicious and nutritious fruits and vegetables to include in your diet. It is certainly not a one-size-fits-all activity, and as you eat them your gut garden will appreciate you. You'll notice your taste buds will also change, becoming enlivened — everything will seem to taste that much richer and your desire for the non-nutritive food like substances (the hyperpalatable processed foods such as the chips, crackers, cookies, snack mixes and bars, breads and other salty or sweet snacks) will significantly diminish. Give these prebiotic treasures a try, and see how your body and gustatory sensory system react to them.

And if you hear the health world buzz with the latest discovery of an exotic food, it doesn't mean it is necessarily right for you. Some people may not do well with certain foods, and that is okay. For instance, nightshade vegetables and fruit such as tomatoes, peppers, eggplant, potatoes, and goji berries all contain lectins. Personally, I am not sensitive to these, and eat many of them in moderation. Yet listening to your body is key here, and I often use the dictum "eat the rainbow," meaning eat a variety of colorful foods – vegetables, and fruit — you enjoy, and to which you don't have a sensitivity.

But, speaking of lectins...

Lectins — Friend or Foe for Your Diet?

I did not bring up lectin-containing nightshades to make you fear them — although, some people seem to be wary of them after recent health enthusiasts popularized potential downsides to eating foods with lectins — or to get into a lengthy discussion on the biochemistry of lectins. I am simply making the point that your diet is YOUR diet, and it should be individualized.

Some people cannot tolerate foods containing certain lectins (lectins are plant proteins that are defense chemicals, and some may even be considered antinutrients), and for those affected by this plant protein, avoidance or limited consumption is advised. The foods I eat containing lectins are members of the nightshade family. I also enjoy legumes and beans (soy, kidney, black beans) as well as sprouted grains (ancient grains, steel-cut oats, et cetera). I try to avoid gluten, not because I have celiac (I don't), but I feel better without it in my diet.

As with fermented foods, those containing lectins are better tolerated when fermented, or also well-cooked — especially pressure-cooked like beans. Furthermore, they could benefit you more if you consumed them sprouted and/or fermented.

I did not find sufficient research to suggest that eliminating lectins entirely from the diet is necessarily the right path though strongly promoted by some. There is, however, significant evidence showing we have been eating them for millennia, many having notable health benefits, like the tomato. Though if you are sensitive, avoid those that cause you trouble. I personally could not live without tomatoes, and thankfully I don't have a problem digesting them. Aside from lectins, tomatoes contain the very beneficial antioxidant lycopene, which has been suggested to reduce rates in prostate cancer.[169]

Diversity is the Spice of Life –
For Us and the Gut

I prefer to take a wide-angle-view approach to observe not only the current environment, but its context, and use the benefit of incorporating our human history into the equation. When I use this approach, one of the biggest issues I see regarding our current nutrition and health is our tendency to eat a very limited number of natural foods that are available to us (replacing many with industrialized processed foods). We simply do not have enough diversity of natural plant and animal foods in our diet, compared to our ancestors. This so-called agrobiodiversity has rapidly and consistently declined year after year, especially in the last 120 years.[170]

For example, it has been estimated that there are approximately 300,000 edible plants, compared with the average humans' consumption of less than 200 of them.[170] Only three of them make up the majority of plant calories in our diet; over half by conservative estimates. Any ideas as to what these three plants are? I am sure you know — corn, wheat, and rice, while coming up quickly in the rearview mirror is soy. Furthermore, it was estimated in 2004 that 75% of the world's food is generated from only twelve plants and five animal species.[171]

Beyond this, according to the Food and Agriculture Organization (FAO) of the United Nations, more than 90% of cultivated crop varieties have disappeared from farmers' fields in recent years, and half of the breeds of many domestic animals have also been lost.[171] This trend is not only a travesty, but it significantly impacts human health *and* that of our microbiota.

Prove me wrong here. Make a list of all the plant foods you regularly eat, vegetables and fruit especially, and see if you can name some different ones that you could eat in any given week. Most of us will have trouble naming fifty overall. I think you get my point. Fortunately, this *can* change, just remember to focus on *adding* more to your diet, the whole rainbow, as we strive to incorporate more diversity both for taste and for health!

Expanding our diet with real whole, natural, and well-sourced unprocessed foods is not only exciting and fun, but beneficial to our overall health, and serves as a direct link to the health of our microbiota. Clearly, we've established that our gut bacteria, our microbiota, like diversity. The saying "diversity is the spice of life" applies here. Eating a broad array of natural whole foods is great for our gut garden!

In fact, a scientific paper proved the merits of diversity for gut health in the peer-reviewed journal *Molecular Metabolism*, dated March of 2016. The authors concluded from the extensive data reviewed that, "The more diverse the diet, the more diverse the microbiome and the more adaptable it will be to perturbations."[172] So, eating a varied diet is not only better for us (humans), but also for them (gut bacteria), while also being beneficial to combating challenges and stressors that may arise.

Unfortunately, this pathway to the diversity of gut health and overall health improvement has been significantly blocked. According to the Food and Agricultural Organization of the United Nations, 75% of plant genetic diversity has been lost.[171] Farmers worldwide have traded their multiple local varieties for the genetically uniform, high-yielding, pesticide-resistant GMO varieties of food, in many cases.

The practices of using genetically modified organisms (GMOs), along with their often associated pesticides — such as the well-known glyphosate used in farming, and antibiotics as growth promoters in raised livestock — BOTH negatively impact our gut microbiota. These practices result in much less diversity, harming many of the beneficial strains of bacteria both in our microbiota and in the host, plant, and animal. Think of pesticide use in plants as similar to antibiotics for animals and humans. Pesticides affect plants' microbiota negatively, just as antibiotics do for animals, us and our gut bacteria.

In many cases, the dysbiosis (disproportionate amount of unhealthy bacteria compared to healthy ones) which occurs in the source food continues in us, the eventual host. In other words, if we eat foods exposed to pesticides or antibiotics during their cultivation, these will ALSO harm us and negatively affect our gut health, via our microbiota.[173] So *we are not only what we eat*, but also what we *eat has eaten* and been exposed to.

Evidence showing the preponderance of antibiotic use in growing many foods we eat (approximately 80% of all antibiotics sold in the U.S. are used for animal agriculture) negatively affects the source and later consumer (us).[174] These effects are present in farm-raised animals as well. Not only do they become obese, and tend to have a less diverse obesogenic microbiome, but when we consume them we ingest the same toxins, limiting our chances for healthy gut microbiota and increasing the chances of weight gain.

I could go on and on here about this worldwide practice. Fortunately, we ultimately decide the fate of this practice, when we "vote with our feet, our wallets, and our *forks*." We can refuse to buy foods cultured and raised with these harmful chemicals and unhealthy practices. They don't help us, our gut microbiome, or the earth, and we can do better. If we steer towards a healthy microbiome and boycott foods that prevent us from achieving gut health, things will have to eventually change. So, make an effort to buy foods that are healthy for your gut and your body — well sourced and organic!

Remember, paying attention to the quality and source of your foods and how they were cultivated, both plant and animal, is key. We are not only what we eat, but what our food has eaten and been exposed to. This can be done at your own pace, and is not an all-or-nothing event. Start by slowly adding well-sourced organic foods to your diet *regularly*!

From my experience with a family of eight, it was initially a bit more expensive to go from "zero to sixty," and start on day one with nothing but organic and well-sourced vegetables and fruit. Try adding a few at a time. It is still more important to buy and consume real whole food, whether organic or not, than to eat a diet rich in highly processed industrialized foods that come in a package.

So adjust your practices little by little, as your budget allows. In the end, it WILL be WORTH it. At the outset, it may seem expensive, but in the end, poor health is much more expensive. Trust me. As a physician for more than two decades, I have seen how the negative effects of poor health can trample one's income, productivity, and enjoyment of life, many times over.

> *You will not regret investing both in quality well-sourced food and your health.*
>
> *I have never seen a person unhappy with the results.*

CHAPTER 9

Foods and Practices that will Enhance Gut Health

"Leave your drugs in the chemist's pot if you can heal the patient with food. . .
Let food be thy medicine, and medicine be thy food."
— **Hippocrates**

While we are on the topic of adding quality foods to the diet, let's continue discussing those that benefit our gut bacteria, their diversity, and the microbiome. In addition to the prebiotic-rich fibrous foods and the fermented ones already mentioned, there are a few others to consider.

You may be wondering if there are any to avoid — YES. Yet I always like to first include the things we should ADD to our diet, and then talk about those to avoid. Ultimately, I think you will be pleasantly surprised with how many *more* there are to *add* than those to *subtract* — those we should avoid all share very simple themes. Don't worry, you won't have to remember any exhaustive list or buy another app, just incorporate a couple of simple rules I will mention.

Additions

Remember, the key is to add a *variety* of real, whole, natural, well-sourced foods, and eliminate those highly processed and the less than ideally raised ones. For example, adding more varieties of:

- Healthy vegetables and fruits (such as berries and grapes [remember the powerful polyphenol antioxidants they have, like resveratrol])
- Cruciferous vegetables (broccoli, cauliflower, cabbage, and Brussels sprouts)
- Leafy greens (spinach, kale, and Swiss chard)
- Artichokes, chickpeas, lentils, green peas
- Nuts like almonds (high in both prebiotic fiber and polyphenols), macadamia, and pistachios
- Garlic
- Ginger
- Cacao
- Healthy cooking oils (especially extra virgin minimally processed olive oil)
- Coconut and MCT oil
- Avocado oil
- Grass-fed butter, ghee, and tallow)
- Healthy wild proteins, such as wild-caught low mercury fish like wild salmon, sardines, and anchovies
- Grass-fed and pasture raised regenerative meats
- And if you tolerate grains, sprouted grains are best.
- Fermented foods as discussed in the last section are super nutritious, healthy and savory!

Now, this is not an exhaustive list, but it gives you a good springboard for foods that are healthy for you and them, and will prove to be a useful aid while maintaining your healthy gut garden.

Now that we know what foods are good for your gut garden, let's briefly summarize the behaviors that will also enhance and optimize your gut health. In addition to eating these gut-healthy foods, getting an appropriate amount of sleep is critical to the health of your microbiota. Just as it was discussed at length in the circadian rhythm chapter, our gut flora ALSO has a circadian clock. It performs best when optimized to the same ancestral day and night cycle in which we operate our daily lives. High-quality sleep cycles will result in tangible benefits to our microbiota too.

In fact, the health of our gut microbiota is directly related to our sleep quality, as demonstrated by Smith and colleagues in their preeminent scientific paper, "Gut microbiome diversity is associated with sleep physiology in humans." They showed that increased sleep efficiency is directly correlated with improved gut health, measured by increased microbial diversity. Poor sleep had the opposite effect.[175]

This study was performed by measuring participants' sleep, recorded by a wearable bio-tracking sleep device. Researchers took stool samples of each participant to study their gut microbiota during a month of sleep monitoring. They found that gut bacteria could directly impact sleep, and vice-versa, likely due to the involvement of the brain-gut-microbiome axis (BGMA). Their findings also suggest that diversity of the gut microbiome promotes healthier sleep.[175] This is an amazing find! We help them by taking care of not only their food, but also our (and their) environment. In addition, they can also help us obtain that "good night's sleep!" Another win-win!

Our Second Brain

Many of you have likely heard of the gut-brain connection, and interestingly it has been shown to significantly impact many aspects of health, far beyond the obvious connection with the gastrointestinal (GI) system. In fact, the microbiota interacting via this BGMA has been shown to affect behavioral and mood disorders such as autism, depression, and anxiety, as well as affecting cognitive functioning and disorders such as Parkinson's and Alzheimer's, both positively or negatively. This depends on the health of the gut microbiota and its diversity.

The connectivity that occurs through both neurotransmitters and signaling molecules produced by the gut bacteria, as well as the signals sent down the vagus nerve from the brain — which has numerous synapses with the brain and the gut. *No, what happens in the vagus does not stay in the vagus.* It has far-reaching consequences, many of which are in the gut. And this can be a really GOOD thing!

In fact, this connection between the brain (central nervous system) and the gut (enteric nervous system) is not only physical and anatomical, but also has metabolic, endocrine, humoral, and immune connectivity! This links the autonomic nervous system (the at ease, rest, and digestive system) to the stress response hormonal system (hypothalamic-pituitary-adrenal axis [HPA]) and the nerves within the gut GI tract (enteric nervous plexus) to both the gut and the brain.

This allows the bidirectional influence of the brain on the gut, and vice versa, to affect mood, cognition, and mental health.176 As briefly mentioned previously, this amazing inherent connection and bidirectional process of communication is what leads many to call the gut our "second brain." It is much too powerful to ignore, and its understanding is key to our brain health, as well as that of our emotional, metabolic, and immune systems.

There is now a preponderance of evidence showing this connection between the intestinal microbiota and its profound influence on emotional, cognitive, metabolic, and immune health spheres. For example, the makeup of the gut microbiota and its neurohormonal messengers has been shown to play a role in anxiety, depression, and autism spectrum disorders.

In an exceptional 2020 scientific review, "Gut Microbiome and Depression: How Microbes Affect the Way We Think," the authors delineate numerous pathways involved in the neurohumoral communication (via neurotransmitters like serotonin and dopamine, and hormones like cortisol and epinephrine) between the gut microbiota and the brain, which contribute to mood and brain function. After their extensive review of the available literature, they concluded that indeed there *is* a strong link between the microbes in our gut and how we think.166 Indeed, the gut-brain axis is an essential pathway to consider in the management of brain health and mood disorders.

It has been discovered that, again, the diversity of our gut bacteria plays a key role in brain health. In mood disorders like depression, a decrease in diversity was present, and by specifically targeting the microbiota to improve diversity, a potential treatment option in depression and mood disorders may be promising, as the gut bacteria exert a significant positive influence in mood disorders.[178,179] In other words, making your gut healthy using the prescribed methods above can also be beneficial to your mood. *"Happy gut, happy life"* could be the mantra here!

Appreciating this gut health pearl of knowledge in our current environment is especially empowering. Sadly, during the recent COVID-19 pandemic, it has been found that mood disorders have risen extensively. Anxiety, depression, and PTSD are at levels never-before-seen. According to a recent study published in December of 2020, "The COVID-19 pandemic represents an unprecedented threat to mental health in high, middle, and low-income countries."[180] Therefore, there truly is no time like the present to buff up our gut health for our mood *and* our life!

What many people, including most doctors in my experience, often do not realize is that the majority of serotonin (the "happy" hormone/neurotransmitter), is produced in the gut. Indeed, it has been estimated by researchers Banskota and colleagues that up to 95% of serotonin is in the gut, and only about 5% is found in the brain.[181] No wonder gut health is so important to mental health — it's science!

In addition to diet, sleep, and stress management, which if optimized can all significantly improve the health and diversity of our gut microbiota, it has also been shown that moderate exercise can also carry out a protective role in gut health. Exercise enriches the microflora diversity, and can improve the *Bacteroidetes: Firmicutes* ratio, which may contribute to reducing weight and obesity-associated health conditions.[182]

Daily movement is key to optimizing your overall health *and* that of your gut microbiota. Now, as mentioned in the chapter on movement, it can occasionally be overdone by chronic over-exercising. This is rare, but in this case your gut can be adversely affected due to excessive stress and the overactivation of cortisol and the HPA (hypothalamic-pituitary-adrenal) axis.

Have you ever run a marathon or a similarly long race or distance? Ever wonder why you may have gotten some GI upset? Excessive running with the associated stress may be the issue. You may be overdoing it by running long distances too often, or performing any chronic single sport exercise excessively, which can cause stress on the body and the gut. However, the more common problem is the lack of sufficient exercise in the developed world.

> *We are in the driver's seat,*
> *so we can change this.*

CHAPTER 10

Habits that Hurt the Gut:
The Gut "Wreckers"

> *"Take care of your body.*
> *It's the only place you have to live."*
> **–Jim Rohn**

Now that we have touched upon a few powerful things that can help to optimize our gut health and its connection to our brain and mental health, let's explore some critical habits to AVOID; those that can negatively impact our gut health and diversity. I often refer to these as the "Gut Wreckers," and will now provide a short yet important list of these gut wreckers we should try to avoid.

Things to avoid:

- Antibiotics
- Antacids
- NSAIDS (Non-steroidal anti-inflammatory drugs) like ibuprofen
- Alcohol
- Poor diet
- A sedentary lifestyle
- Smoking
- Too little sleep

- Stress
- Overuse of "hygiene" products (hand sanitizers and chemical soaps, shampoos, and cosmetics)

To understand the impact of the common "gut wreckers" many of us have been exposed to, let's look at an example — the plight of one of my relatives, whom we will call Daniel. When Daniel was born, his mother developed a fever during the interim of childbirth, so he was placed on a course of intravenous antibiotics within the first days of his life. During his toddler years, Daniel seemed to develop common respiratory illnesses with a cough and fever, and even ear pain numerous times.

By the time he was five years old, Daniel, not unlike many children, had already been on more than half a dozen courses of antibiotics. He then developed "stomach issues," such as crampy abdominal pains, that would often keep him up at night, so bad they warranted late-night hospital visits. The testing that was done there, from abdominal imaging to blood work, always seemed "fine," and this was even more frustrating to his parents, as "no one could find anything wrong." Yet they knew something was not quite right.

He continued to struggle with bloating, stomach pains, and constipation. He even began losing weight, because his stomach hurt so often that he did not have much of an appetite. He had been placed on a variety of over-the-counter and prescription medications, such as acid reducers, stool softeners, and many potent constipation remedies. Yet still his health did not seem to improve.

I listened intently to his mother, as this was severely affecting her son and their family. And ultimately, we decided to make some dietary changes to rebuild his gut. Given I was made aware of the multiple courses of antibiotics he had been exposed to, and the likely significant toll this had taken on his gut, I was hopeful this method would become a major source of relief for Daniel.

We used the seed, feed, and weed approach to rebuild his gut microbiota. After removing much of the processed foods (the generally white and bland colored foods found in the center of most grocery stores), we added probiotic-rich foods such as yogurt, kefir, and kimchi, as well as probiotic supplements. The prebiotic-rich fiber in his diet was also increased. We did this by adding more whole foods, including fresh fruits, vegetables, and legumes. Organic apples, bananas, black beans, asparagus, and even seaweed were also easily added to his diet, while processed foods like the breakfast cereals, crackers, cookies, and chips he used to consume were left out.

Within a few months, not only was he no longer suffering from abdominal pains, but his appetite, bowel movements, and weight had all improved. This was accomplished simply with a food-first approach, giving special attention to foods that would improve his gut health.

The Antibiotic Assault

As a physician, I have witnessed first-hand the overuse of antibiotics. It is an embarrassing fact of which the majority of practicing physicians are guilty. We must do better; the health of our microbiota depends on physician discretion in prescribing antibiotics.

If you are not a physician — the very people to whom I write this book, I presume the majority are not — and your health care provider recommends antibiotics, simply ask if antibiotics are absolutely necessary to treat your condition. In my experience, many antibiotics are unnecessarily prescribed.

The CDC reports that as many as one in three prescriptions for antibiotics are deemed "unnecessary."[183] Working in medicine for over twenty years, I regard this as quite a conservative statistic. The true number is likely higher. In common cases of sinusitis and bronchitis, in which the etiology or cause is overwhelmingly viral, it means that antibiotics are unnecessary as they do not help resolve viral illnesses.

Yet many patients in these cases are still given an antibiotic prescription. To cement this fact, the AAFP (American Academy of Family Physicians) found that more than eighty percent of health care visits from adults and children for sinusitis resulted in antibiotic prescriptions.[184] The very case I just shared related to one boy's experience with multiple, likely unnecessary, courses of antibiotics ultimately affecting his health and gut.

As physicians, we can do better and use antibiotics more discriminately. They can be life-saving, so why not save them for when they are truly needed? Overuse can not only potentially cause "super bacteria" with antibiotic resistance, but it also may have significant detrimental consequences to our gut microbiota.

According to a scientific review on this topic, to cite once again, the *British Medical Journal* in September of 2020, which included 31 scientific papers, it was determined that antibiotics commonly used in primary care settings showed a rapid impact on the gut microbiota: decreased commensal bacterial levels and decreased diversity of gut bacteria, which causes the gut microbiota to take several weeks to six months to recover after a single course.[185]

Remember that decreasing the diversity of our gut microbiota is a sign of poor gut health and puts us at risk for many problems. Antibiotic use has been implicated in decreased gut diversity, and selection for more pathogenic strains such as *C. Difficile, S. Typhimurium,* and Enterohemorrhagic *E. Coli,* which can all cause devastating and even life-threatening intestinal diseases, such as hemorrhagic colitis. Decreased gut diversity has also been shown to adversely affect the immune system, by negatively impacting our ability to fight disease and by potentially contributing to allergies and autoimmune conditions.[208]

Yet this is still not all. Antibiotics have also been shown to contribute to the dysbiosis that leads to insulin resistance and obesity.[186] I think you get the picture.

Avoid unnecessary antibiotic use, and both your body and gut will thank you.

A Sedentary Life Stunts Your
Gut Health and Your Lifespan

Next on the list is a lifestyle choice to avoid: the far too common sedentary trap that wrecks our gut. I have found that a mostly inactive lifestyle can easily creep up on any of us and quickly become that path of least resistance, *if* we don't proactively consider alternatives. Remember earlier in the book, we spoke of metabolism, and how there is a common misconception that our metabolism slows with age? Many of us, including me, have blamed calendar years on what appears to be a slowing metabolism that ultimately leads to weight gain.

However, research shows, just as I have elucidated in this book thus far, that at least until we are sixty years old, our metabolism does *not* significantly slow down.[41] What changes is us; *we change.* Our activity levels and dietary choices are likely to blame. Now, I know this may not be a fact you wanted to hear. Nevertheless, it is true.

The flip side of this revelation is that *we* are in control of this! *We* decide our activity levels, and what ends up at the end of our fork. *We* have the power to choose a better way of living.

To emphasize the unhealthy magnitude of this sedentary curse on modern health, we like to say, in the health and wellness sphere, that sitting is the new smoking. The data shows that a sedentary lifestyle is strongly associated with the leading causes of death — heart disease, cancer, diabetes —

and correlates with premature death.[187] Indeed, total daily sedentary hours and television viewing time directly correlated with an increase in all-cause mortality risk.[188] No matter what our health history, predisposition, or overall health status is, increased inactivity (sitting) is a risk factor for dying. Simply stated, the more we sit, the quicker we die.

It appears as though the average person in recent years spends the majority of their day in sedentary positions, and this is *not* awesome. Sitting at a computer, behind the wheel of a car, at a desk, or watching TV or Netflix — whatever the scenario may be. From my observation, this has only gotten worse since the effects of COVID-19 forced closures of schools and businesses, mandatory quarantines, and so on. In fact, knowing the correlation between sedentary behavior and an earlier death, I wrote the majority of this book standing at my improvised standing desk — made by placing a cardboard box on a table or my kitchen counter to raise the height. It's the simple things!

Being sedentary is not good for us or our gut, both literally and figuratively. Our gut flora also respond to this "action" of non-activity. One study has shown that increased sedentary behavior is correlated to decreased diversity in the gut flora, and that exercise can increase beneficial strains of gut bacteria, such as the health-promoting bacterial species: *Faecalibacterium prausnitzii, Roseburia hominis,* and *Akkermansia muciniphila.* The increase in these healthy strains of bacteria in this study appeared to be independent of diet. In other words, exercise alone exerted a positive microbiota effect, separate from diet. The groups in this study had a similar dietary makeup, and differed predominantly in exercise patterns.[189] Thus, another reason to *get up and move.*

Fortunately, despite the near direct dose-response correlation of increased sitting on mortality (more sitting time directly proportional to increased premature mortality), these negative mortality effects of sitting were effectively erased when moderate to vigorous physical activity at recommended intervals (150–299 minutes a week) was inserted into the picture, according to a study in the *Journal of the American College of Cardiology.*[188] As little as thirty minutes a day, five days a week, did the trick.

Translation: this can be done easily with a simple 30-minute walk each day.

Movement for the win!

Poor Sleep Damages the Gut

Sleep is critical to acquiring and maintaining optimal gut health. Like nearly every living thing, our microbiota also respond to sleep-wake cycles, and are affected by perturbations in them. Both fragmented sleep and short sleep duration are associated with gut dysbiosis, which impacts our health and our gut in many negative ways.

It is a fact that some of the metabolic disturbances associated with sleep loss may be mediated through the overgrowth of specific gut bacteria. Their signaling across the established neurohumoral pathways of the gut-brain axis may affect our behaviors via hormones and other signaling pathways. Li and colleagues, in their review article on sleep and the microbiome in the scientific journal *Frontiers in Psychiatry*, suggest that circadian misalignment and sleep loss in humans are associated with dysbiosis, and that the resulting microbiota shifts may contribute to metabolic imbalances.[190]

They further explain that these resulting microbiota shifts cause inflammation, metabolic disorders, and even impaired immune function. Furthermore, this process ultimately changes the metabolism of communicating neurotransmitters, resulting in nervous system dysfunction such as sleep disruptions, or even psychiatric symptoms — starting a vicious cycle.[191]

In other words, sleep and the microbiome are intimately intertwined, and it is paramount to safeguard our sleep and stick to a solid circadian cycle. Without good sleep, we may suffer gut dysbiosis, metabolic disorders such as insulin resistance, obesity, and diabetes, and settle into a proinflammatory state. In turn, this can make us become more susceptible to not only infection with a compromised immune system, but to many chronic diseases. Taken together, this also puts us at risk for mental health challenges such as depression, anxiety, and other mental health concerns.

For example, take the case of my wife, who like me is in her forties. She got to a point in her health regime where she became concerned that her metabolism was slowing. Despite her six or seven days a week exercise routine and eating a clean diet of real foods, she struggled with getting that stubborn last 5–10 pounds to melt away. What we found was that quality and sufficient sleep was the one thing lacking in her approach. Her diet, exercise, stress optimization, and gut health were all given heavy focus, but her sleep was not. Once she dialed into a solid seven to eight-hour nightly regimen and prioritized this daily, the magic started to happen. The remaining few pounds were lost, and the only change was safeguarding her sleep!

Prioritizing sleep is something we just can't afford to skimp on. The "sleep when we're dead" mantra that I used to subscribe to just doesn't work. Safeguarding our sleep will not only benefit us, but also the microbiota, which will in turn provide us with even more benefits. The stress response that gets triggered by decreased or fragmented sleep can initiate a cascade of inflammation.

This associated signaling between the gut and the brain triggers dysbiosis, favoring species that can further derange our hormones. This will ultimately affect our metabolism, leading to insulin resistance, weight gain, and even mood disorders such as depression and anxiety.

> **Sleep CAN and NEEDS to be one of our SUPERPOWERS.**

Knowing, as they say, is at best only half the battle, and doing is what really moves the needle. Feel free to revisit and re-read the chapter on circadian rhythm and sleep, in order to make the most of this extremely potent tool, and get the gut and body synced for success. You've got this! Don't wait to sleep when you're dead!

Stress Ruins the Gut

Stress, as we have touched upon, is not only potentially detrimental to us but also our gut microbiota. This connection has been increasingly studied in recent years, and is becoming more recognized and appreciated. Deep connections are being discovered between the stress response and the gut microbiota, ultimately affecting the makeup of the bacterial species as well as the immune function.

It can affect their response to stress hormones like cortisol and adrenaline, but also have possible effects on the body's response to and formation of visceral pain.[192] It is now generally understood that an overactive or repeated stress response (fight or flight sympathetic response) ultimately leads to dysbiosis, decreased immune function, and leaky gut.

It may also contribute to pathologic bacterial colonization and ongoing inflammation, contributing to many chronic diseases. This is the maladaptive stress or negative stress referred to in the previous chapter, not the more beneficial challenge response phenomenon which we should strive to adopt.

Choosing to respond to stress as a challenge, instead of receiving it as a threat, likely has more beneficial effects, as discussed previously, through the oxytocin effect and other positive signaling pathways. Resulting from our positive mindset and how we choose to respond to stress also determines how our microbiota react.

A new study published in September 2021 looked at oxytocin and its effects on the microbiome of rats that were subjected to the stress hormone analog of cortisol. What they found was that oxytocin, the same hormone that is released in the human body in the adaptive challenge response, positively shifted the rat microbiota to one having more of the genus *Mogibacterium,* which is associated with low anxiety behavior in rats.[193]

Although this was a rat study, the results are very exciting as they give more evidence of the strong and far-reaching effects of the beneficial hormone, oxytocin, which is released when we choose to respond to stress as a challenge, and not a threat. These beneficial effects of oxytocin are not only felt in calming our nerves, but are as far-reaching as our gut microbiota!

This is groundbreaking!

> *We all will have stress at some time or another,*
> *but the key element is CHOICE.*
> *We can choose how we respond to it.*
> *And that very choice may just make all the difference.*

Over-Sanitation and Hygiene Products
May Ruin the Gut

Rounding out this section on "gut wreckers," I'll briefly touch on the ill effects to our microbiota that pervasive use of hygiene products can pose. It is well known that hand sanitizers and certain hygiene products can affect the skin and gut microbiota, but overuse can seriously damage our microbial flora, and encourage growth of pathogenic and resistant strains. Recently this has become an even greater concern due to the widespread and frequent sanitization practices that have escalated during the recent years of COVID-19.

I share a similar concern to the reputable Dr. A. Singh, a renowned scientist and professor, who wrote in the *British Medical Journal* about his heightened concern of the "immeasurable effect of the large scale use of disinfectants and sanitisers in the COVID-19 pandemic on the microbiomes of various ecological niches in humans, animals, and environments. Dysbiosis in host-commensal interactions is a likely outcome of such practices, thereby affecting the host's immune functioning, metabolism, physiological parameters, and susceptibility to infectious and non-infectious diseases."[194]

The increases in use are well known, and the patterns of antibiotic resistance and damage to our microbiota are only now starting to become appreciated. As we navigate the world of sanitizers and disinfectants and their uses as a society, we should remember to consider the collateral damages of such practices to us and our microbiota, and seek to use them in appropriate scenarios with caution. We must, then, consider potential downstream effects and how to best minimize them.

It is also very interesting to me that, historically, overuse of antibiotics and over-sanitization in the industrialized world have likely led to increased issues with allergy, immune, and autoimmune diseases than ever before. The perturbation of our microbiome through the overuse of "sanitization" practices is quite disturbing.

Now, I am not saying that it's not good to wash your hands prior to performing surgery, or any medical procedure for that matter, or to take antibiotics for certain infections; these are, of course, important practices and potentially life-saving remedies. But I *am* saying that over the years, and especially of late, we may have become too comfortable overdoing it.

As a society, we may also be forgetting some
important yet simple practices our ancestors
did for millennia, which strengthened their microbiomes:
walking barefoot, eating organic (pesticide-free)
and wild or self-grown fruits and vegetables, and
raising livestock without the industrialized
practices of antibiotics and hormone use.

A deeper dive into these important topics can be found in the books: *The Microbiome Solution* (2015) by Dr. Robynne Chutkan and *Food Fix* (2020) by Dr. Mark Hyman. These penned contributions are great reads, and I recommend them both for more information on these critical topics.

In addition to the over sterilization that may occur with the overuse of hand sanitizers, antibiotics, and hygiene products (please visit the very informative ewg.org website of the *Environmental Working Group*, which is a great resource for information on the safety of food and cosmetic products), many common and over-the-counter (OTC) medications also have the potential to wreck the microbiome.

Common OTC Meds Can Impair The Gut

Unfortunately, most people, even many doctors, are not aware of this common unintended consequence of over-the-counter (OTC) medication. For example, commonly used antacid/heartburn relief medications, like the PPI (proton pump inhibitor) class of OTC medications — such as lansoprazole (Prevacid), esomeprazole (Nexium), and omeprazole (Prilosec) — are one of the most commonly used pharmaceutical classes in the world, and consistently rank top 10 in both non-prescription and prescription medication sold.

While instructions may indicate use for a brief specified amount of time, these drugs are unfortunately often taken indiscriminately, and for longer periods, by consumers who are unaware of the potentially devastating side effects to their digestion and microbiome. Though generally regarded as safe, and available without a prescription, these OTC medications literally have the capacity to quickly and powerfully derange the gut microbiota.

This manifests by decreasing the natural pH (lowering the acidity levels which helps the good bacteria fight invading pathogens) of the GI tract, making us more prone to pathogenic organisms and dysbiosis. They also decrease the efficiency of our food absorption and metabolism (like decreasing the absorption of vitamin B12, for example).

In a recent study published in the scientific journal *Gut*, Imhann and colleagues discuss significantly negative and deleterious effects of this extremely common medication class, evaluated in their study of 1,815 patients. What they found was that the PPI class (proton pump inhibitor antacids, described above) caused a much less healthy gut microbiome, susceptible to bacterial overgrowth, dysbiosis, and more facile infection.[195]

These shifts in bacteria are known to predispose individuals taking PPIs to the dreaded C. *difficile* colitis infections, as well as cause an increased risk of other enteric infections in PPI users. They made the strong conclusion that, on a population level, the effects of the PPI class of antacid medications are more prominent and profound than the effects of antibiotics, or other commonly used drugs, on the microbiome.[195] This is a very bold statement to make, but it highlights the importance of exercising caution with antacids as well as other "gut wreckers" typically regarded as safe.

Next time you consider reaching for an antacid, especially those readily available in the PPI class, consider other options. Start with contemplating the underlying cause of the symptoms in the first place, and consider a natural remedy. Masking the symptoms with an antacid does not address the underlying cause, and carries the possibility of significant side effects on the gut microbiome, which is not a healthy option.

In fact, a large analysis directly observed the prevalence of vitamin B12 deficiency among people who regularly take antacid medication. In this large trial of 20,000 patients, with over 4,000 having vitamin B12 deficiency, they discovered those taking acid-lowering medication on a regular basis had a significantly increased incidence of Vitamin B12 deficiency. This presents a serious issue, and without treatment can cause severe neurologic consequences.[196]

The effects of OTC and prescription medications in relation to the gut microbiome have been implicated in other studies as well. Vila and colleagues studied the effects of various common medications on the gut microbiome, and reported that of those they studied, fifteen different medication types created consistent increases in antibiotic resistance genes in those taking them, compared to participants who did not.[197] In other words, more than a dozen classes of medications other than antibiotics and acid-lowering medications caused the increased potential for antibiotic resistance.

In another study looking at the effect of common medications prescribed, and their effects on the microbiome, Jackson and colleagues found that nineteen of the fifty-two prescription medications they studied had a significant correlation to negative effects on the gut microbiome.[198] Nearly half of them! This tells me that any medication may be suspect in wreaking havoc on the microbiome, and we should all be aware of this possibility. (Note — the research is still young here, and likely with time more information on the interaction between medications and the gut microbiome will solidify.)

Indeed, more data is needed in this area, as the research is new and limited, but I believe there has been enough presented so far to inspire in us a desire to learn more about the medication, food, drink, and practices we have adopted, and consider their effects on our microbiome, our "gut garden."

The moral of this story is at least two-fold. First, never assume that just because a medication is prescribed by your doctor, or available over the counter without a prescription, it is safe or can be taken without significant side effects. *Like with food, READ THE LABEL and become familiar with the data!*

Second, in my experience, I have found it generally better practice to *treat the underlying cause* of the symptoms or disease from a root cause approach, than a simple reductionist symptom approach through medication. In other words, simply prescribing or taking medication to treat a specific symptom of an underlying problem or disease without treating the root cause may mask the real issue. It also sets the stage to ignore potentially significant side effects.

I do not believe "bandage" or superficial symptom-based prescription medical treatment is necessarily the answer. Locating the *root cause* from a functional and integrative approach, and then addressing it, is more likely to yield superior and longer-lasting treatment results.

I've adopted a *prevention over prescription* approach.

When it comes down to it, the simple principles and approaches to health you have learned in this book will put you in a good place to continue your journey towards significantly improving your health, waistline, and life. Not only is it simple, but both possible and doable for each of us!

You are now armed with the information — all you have to do is incorporate it into your life, one step at a time. And if you do so, positive health-promoting results are likely in your future!

You've got this!

Alcohol and Smoking Can Damage Your Gut

It should not be surprising that alcohol and smoking are harmful to human health, and by extension to our gut microbiota. Alcohol use causes a decline in the protective gut flora that has anti-inflammatory activity, and puts us at risk for dysbiosis and leaky gut. It also predisposes us to GI cancers, such as gastric cancer.[199]

Unsurprisingly, smoking also has harmful effects on the gut microbiota. The oxidative stress from smoking leads to alterations in the tight junctions and mucin production, causing a leaky gut, while also decreasing the diversity of species, leading to dysbiosis. Interestingly, the inflammatory state of the intestinal tract as a result of smoking closely resembles that of the inflammatory bowel disorder Crohn's disease, which as you can guess, is not a good thing.[200]

In addition to their inflammatory nature, smoking and alcohol use also lead to decreased diversity in the gut. The good news is this can be quickly modified, with smoking cessation.

You CAN change this, and can do so now.

A recent study published in 2020 in the *Journal of Clinical Medicine* showed how quitting smoking can lead to *rapid* improvements in gut health, blood pressure, heart rate, and inflammatory markers. Sublette and colleagues reported that in a 12-week smoking cessation trial, the bacterial alpha diversity increased, and the *Bacteroidetes* to *Firmicutes* ratio improved, as did heart rate, blood pressure, and the inflammatory marker C reactive protein (CRP)[201] Thus, despite the negative effects of smoking, these can be modified and improved with cessation in a moderate amount of time. But if you don't want your gut flora "lit," don't light up.

One of the most important aspects of obtaining and maintaining a healthy gut garden is what we FEED it. Above, we discussed the important things to include in our diet, that we need to SEED (probiotic-rich, fermented foods, and then supplement as needed) and FEED (prebiotic-rich fibrous foods) our gut garden.

Next, we will discuss foods to AVOID, which can WRECK our gut. The dominant feature of the SAD or Western diet is that it is heavily based on processed foods, with simple refined carbohydrates, and vegetable seed oils. And as you can imagine, with the information already given up to this point, a diet such as this has been shown to significantly and negatively impact gut health.

What to Feed and Not Feed Your Gut

This notion has been especially impactful to those immigrating to the U.S. from other countries who have adopted the Western diet. This type of diet with a high percentage of highly processed foods has negatively affected their gut health by decreasing microbial diversity and increasing weight.[202]

A 2019 review article published in *Nutrients* reported that a highly processed foods diet wreaks havoc on the gut microbiota, especially the ultra-processed foods such as snack foods and soft drinks — those which commonly contain refined, highly processed grains, flours and sugars, as well as seed oils, artificial sweeteners, colors, and emulsifiers. This leads to dysbiosis, and causes significant inflammation.[203]

Let me give you an example of a friend of mine, whom we will call John, who came to the U.S. with his family from Iran at twelve years old. When he arrived, he was healthy, fit, and had no notable health or gut issues. As he adopted the Western/SAD diet, however (his favorite meal being from one of the best-known fast-food chains selling primarily burgers and fries), he began to suffer from serious gut health issues. He was ultimately diagnosed with Crohn's Disease — a type of inflammatory bowel disease — that was not common in his home country, and absent from his entire family pedigree. He was the first to get it.

Unfortunately, his physicians and health care team did not make the connections between his new diet and his deteriorating health. He continuously suffered from the disease, enduring multiple surgeries and even bowel resections. Taking the matter of his health seriously, he finally remedied his ailments through diet change.

By modifying his eating habits, John was able to prioritize his gut health, change the outcome of his disease, and improve his life overall. No traditional medicine or treatment ever got him as healthy as he then became, by pursuing a natural root cause protocol, whereby he followed similar dietary and gut health strategies to those shared in this book.

Sadly, it has been estimated by Steele and colleagues, who published a landmark paper in the *British Medical Journal* (that you will have become very familiar with!), that in the U.S., 57.9% of our dietary energy intake is in this ultra-processed food category.[204] Not only processed, but ULTRA-processed. This is alarming. Even worse, our children have *more than 67%* of their diet from these ultra-processed inflammatory foods![136] Moreover, it is another reason why I was motivated to write this book!

My hope is that sharing the information herein will serve as a wake-up call as to the extent we are allowing these low-quality, nutrient-depleted, calorically dense foods to affect our overall well-being, and more extensively our gut health. You must understand that these foods not only put us at risk for the obesity track (obesity trends are at an all-time high in the U.S., and worldwide, and only projected to continue) but numerous inflammatory diseases, heart disease (the number one world-wide killer), stroke, cancer, and more.

> We CAN and MUST do more to
> better feed ourselves and our gut.
> Again, it is not only our health
> that is affected by our diet,
> but also that of our microbiota
> — we are also feeding them.

Depending on how we feed them, they can either symbiotically and synergistically help us improve our health, or the converse. Ultimately, it is *our* choice and rests *at the end of our fork.*

In 2018, returning once more to the scientific journal *Nutrients*, Zinocker and Lindseth published an excellent review on how the diet and microbiome interact, and the role of this interaction in metabolic disease. Here, they summarized the negative effects of the ultra-processed foods and their constituents (from the additives like emulsifiers and artificial sweeteners) to the acellular, mostly carbohydrate base that unfortunately makes up the majority of the Western Diet.[137]

These effects were suggested to be disease-causing through their effects on decreasing diversity and promoting an unhealthful micro-bacterial makeup, dysbiosis, and their inflammation-causing properties.[137] This resulting inflammation caused by the Western diet promotes many diverse forms of inflammatory diseases, as mentioned above.

However, you need not worry.

Because yes! *We can change this.* And this starts with the knowledge you are gaining now of what feeds our gut garden best, and by avoiding those highly processed foods with acellular highly processed grains, flours, sugars, and vegetable seed oils, all of which contain unhealthy additives. Though these are calorically dense, they are NUTRIENT POOR foods.

Almost anything we can find at a supermarket that comes in packaging with a label and a barcode is a potential suspect in the ultra processed category. Remember to READ the labels, avoid these highly processed foods (refer back to the pantry purge exercise in the book), and focus on high-quality, well-sourced natural whole foods.

Do this, and both your gut bacteria and body will thank you.

CHAPTER 11

Conclusion — Putting It All Together

> "He who has health has hope,
> and he who has hope has everything."
> – Thomas Carlyle

CONGRATULATIONS!

You have now completed what I hope to have been an incredibly powerful journey, through the principles that I have gleaned in over two decades of study, practice, and application as a fellow health enthusiast and physician.

You must now realize that you *have* the ability and power within you to make the necessary and appropriate positive changes in your health and your life, for the present and your future. This will edge you forward in your journey towards optimal health.

Everything you need is already there, *within you.*
You are not broken, and you can do this!

I have constantly seen people just like you succeed by applying these simple strategic steps to achieve the health of their dreams, by incorporating these healthy principles and practices into their lives, and I know *you can do this too.*

You now have the framework to enable you to do so, with the extremely powerful health principles that I have personally witnessed transform my own life, my family's, and thousands of others. And I know you will find joy, fulfillment, and better health through applying these concepts.

Feel free to share the good word with your family, friends, and loved ones as these principles can help anyone who desires better health. And, if you practice them in community, not only will you more likely persist in them and achieve the results you desire, but the unshakeable power of connection will empower both you and those you relate and connect with. Remember we are better together and having an accountability partner or two is great for you and them! And, it is often more fun too!

I have purposely kept the action plans simple, doable, and largely inexpensive (most even free), so that they can be shared and applied to millions of lives, or better yet *billions*, across the globe!

Our good health BEGINS in the gut, and the foundational principles discussed in this book, as summarized below, will carry you far in your pursuit of energy, vitality, and a healthier, and perhaps longer life:

1. FOOD FIRST

Food is the best and most frequent medicine for ourselves, our metabolism, and our gut microbiota.

As we focus on a REAL foods mantra, paying attention to the source and quality of our largely single ingredient whole food, optimizing the TIMING of our food, reducing or eliminating most snacking, and incorporating some version of intermittent or circadian fasting, we CAN be both vibrant and unstoppable.

2. MOVEMENT

Making daily movement a *must* will invigorate you today and for the future, with more energy and focus in the now, as well as a higher performing metabolism, decreasing your risk of encountering a myriad of diseases. Remember, no gym membership or fancy weight set is required here. You can do this simply and sustainably, with your own body and the nature that surrounds you. It can be as simple as converting your desk to a standing one and going for a walk, or two daily! Don't forget the importance of resistance training, strength and balance work with your own body weight through the myriad of easily done at-home body-weight exercises. It *can* be this simple!

3. SLEEP

Safeguarding and supercharging your sleep for both immediate and lifelong benefits will positively affect you and your gut. This simple yet powerful tool cannot be underestimated, and may be that missing ingredient to unleash the potent life force capable of propelling you forward, to succeed with your health and life goals. Plus, it may just help you be a nicer, kinder, and more energetic human, as it did me. Don't wait to "sleep when you're dead" and take advantage of this potent, free, and life-changing tool now!

4. STRESS OPTIMIZATION

Optimizing the stress in your life, your response, and the meaning you attach to it, may be that missing link to balance your hormones and your life. Remember, only *you* can decide what meaning to attach to it, and how to view and respond to the stress that will come your way. The stress will come, but YOU are in charge. *Life happens for you and not to you.* Never forget — you've got this!

5. GUT ENHANCEMENT

And, finally, when we are able to create a happy gut, our lives become so much richer. As we optimize this powerful partnership of our second brain with the powerful neural and hormonal gut feeling, this can lead us along in our path to optimal health. Partnering with your microbiota is a team you definitely want to be a part of as it may be that game changer for your health and your life. It is that important! *Remember, all health begins in the gut!*

I truly believe learning these principles, and then most importantly of all, putting them into *action*, will positively affect your health and your life. I encourage you to re-read them often, share them, and continue to apply the action steps put forward throughout, as you progress into your beautiful new life.

The power of these simple daily practices,
when done consistently,
will keep you on the path towards UNSHAKEABLE health!
You can do this — I am right there with you!

To your health!

Thomas Hemingway, MD

NEXT STEPS

I would love to hear from you! Feel free to tag me in your posts **@drthomashemingway** on Instagram and I'll be happy to read and share them too!

Also, please sign up for my free weekly health pearls newsletter, *"Thursdays to Thrive,"* for ongoing health information and action steps to magnify your health and your life! You can find the link on my website, **https://www.thomashemingway.com**

For updated free weekly content on how to *build unshakeable health*, be sure to subscribe and listen to my weekly **podcast**, anywhere podcasts are found, **The Unshakeable Health Podcast with Thomas Hemingway, M.D.** where I share the most up-to-date and powerful health content to level-up your health and your life!

It would also be my pleasure and joy to have you in the **THRIVE VIP** Community, where you can link arms with like-minded health enthusiasts, and get *exclusive content* and *live webinars*:

https://thomashemingway.podia.com/thomas-hemingway-community

And Deep dive Masterclass Courses Available at:
https://thomashemingway.podia.com

Topics include:
- Natural Weight Loss
- Optimizing Sleep
- Metabolism Reset
- Stress Optimization
- Gut Health Masterclass
- The Magic of Movement (Exercise)
- Intermittent Fasting

And MORE on the WAY!

More with Dr. Thomas Hemingway:

Website: **https://www.thomashemingway.com**

Instagram: **@drthomashemingway**
https://www.instagram.com/drthomashemingway/

Facebook: **Thomas Hemingway MD**
https://www.facebook.com/thomashemingwaymd

LinkedIn: **Thomas Hemingway, MD**
https://www.linkedin.com/in/drthomashemingway

Linktree: **drthomashemingway**
https://linktr.ee/drthomashemingway

Twitter: @doc_hemingway
https://twitter.com/doc_hemingway

Podcast: **Unshakeable Health with Thomas Hemingway, M.D.**

**AND, don't forget to grab your FREE PDF with the ACTION STEPS and SUMMARY of the 5 Powerful Practices described in this book, which can be found on my website: https://www.thomashemingway.com

About the Author

Thomas Hemingway M.D. is a board certified physician, with a special interest in holistic and integrative medicine, who lives and shares his personal and professional philosophy of *prevention over prescription*. He is passionate about sharing the message of an *achievable natural health and healing process*, through *simple* yet *powerful* practices which are doable, and can be life-saving.

He graduated from the University of California, San Diego School of Medicine in 2002, with a Doctor of Medicine Degree, before completing a residency in Emergency Medicine at the University of California, Los Angeles in 2006.

He received his Board Certification from the American Board of Emergency Medicine (ABEM) in 2007, and continues to be board certified with medical licenses in various states including Florida, Hawaii, Utah, and California.

With more than two decades of experience as a physician, he is skilled at making complex health topics understandable and actionable. His primary goal is to save 100 million lives, by optimizing health and wellness through natural means. You can find more of this powerful and actionable message on his weekly podcast **_Unshakeable Health,_** where he breaks down the latest medical knowledge and science into easily digestible and doable steps to help *up-level* your health and your life.

He is also a husband, and proud father to six wonderful humans with whom he enjoys spending time outdoors getting his favorite vitamins, C, M, N, D, and G, (connection, movement, nature, sunshine, and gratitude) while surfing, snowboarding, skiing, biking, hiking, skateboarding, mountaineering, and playing tennis while spending time connecting with those he loves in the great outdoors.

Acknowledgements

I want to take a moment to acknowledge the many wonderful people who in so many ways helped with bringing this important work to life.

Firstly, I **thank God**, for the gift of life and the beautiful, capable, wonderful human body with which I was bestowed — one that can experience so many things, and is innately capable of so much more than we know; *if* we honor it as the magnificent and wonderful creation that it is. Going back to our natural roots, to natural means, and through natural foods and practices which transcend time, can not only strengthen our physiology but also allow us to go and do so many great things as we serve others and fulfill our *ikigai*, or mission.

To **my wife Brooke**, for being my partner in all things, for your endless support, belief, and your amazing gifts of love, patience, and encouragement as we've been on this amazing journey called life, with our beautiful family of six wonderfully energetic children. Thank you for keeping me grounded, connected, and focused with your example and your endless love and support.

To **my children,** who have supported me in every step on this journey to share the life-changing, natural, and holistic health — that has changed our lives forever — with the world. I want to be with each of you for a good, long, vibrant life, and want the same for millions of others. Thank you for always believing in me and for helping me to see how this message needed to get out to the world.

To **my parents,** who have always believed in power through knowledge and corresponding action, and who have believed in and encouraged me to do that which is good, and to share my gifts with the world. Thank you for your support, encouragement, and endless love.

I want to also thank **my tribe at the Unshakeable Health Podcast** who have believed in me and supported me with encouragement and interest as I shared with them along the way many of the messages later incorporated into this book.

I want to thank **Marjah and her team at AWA (Authors Writing Academy)** for helping take hundreds of pages of detailed science-based information and transforming it into a readable book for the masses.

I also want to thank **my patients, friends, family, and followers** both in life and on social media whose continued encouragement kept the flame and desire burning bright to finally get this work out for all to benefit from. Mahalo Nui Loa and Aloha!

To your health!

Thomas Hemingway, MD

References

1- National Center for Chronic Disease Prevention and Health Promotion. "Heart Disease Facts." *CDC*, 14 Oct. 2022, www.cdc.gov/heartdisease/facts.htm. Accessed 1 October 2021

2- Araújo, Joana, et al. "Prevalence of Optimal Metabolic Health in American Adults: National Health and Nutrition Examination Survey 2009–2016." *Metabolic Syndrome and Related Disorders*, vol. 17, no. 1, 2019, pp. 46–52, https://doi.org/10.1089/met.2018.0105.

3- Arias, Elizabeth . "United States Life Tables, 2017." *National Vital Statistics Reports*, vol. 69, no. 7, 2019, https://stacks.cdc.gov/view/cdc/79487.

4- "The Big Number: 45 Million Americans Go on a Diet Each Year: 70 Percent of Adults Are Overweight or Obese, Which Can Lead to Serious Health Problems." *The Washington Post*, 2017.

5- Martin, Crescent, et al. "Attempts to Lose Weight Among Adults in the United States, 2013–2016." *CDC*, Jul. 2018, www.cdc.gov/nchs/products/databriefs/db313.htm.

6- Anderson, James, and Kathleen Abrahamson, Kathleen . "Your Health Care May Kill You: Medical Errors." *Studies in Health Technology and Informatics*, vol. 234, 2017, pp. 13–17, https://doi.org/10.3233/978-1-61499-742-9-13.

7- North, Michael. "Greek Medicine." *National Library of Medicine*, www.nlm.nih.gov/hmd/greek/greek_oath.html. Accessed 20 Apr. 2021.

8 - "Comparison of Dietary Macronutrient Patterns of 14 Popular Named Dietary Programmes for Weight and Cardiovascular Risk Factor Reduction in Adults: Systematic Review and Network Meta-Analysis of Randomised Trials." *BMJ*, vol. 370, 2020, pp. m3095–m3095, https://doi.org/10.1136/bmj.m3095.

9 - Hall, Kevin D., and Scott Kahan. "Maintenance of Lost Weight and Long-Term Management of Obesity." *The Medical Clinics of North America*, vol. 102, no. 1, 2018, pp. 183–97, https://doi.org/10.1016/j.mcna.2017.08.012.

10 - Research and Markets. "United States Weight Loss & Diet Control Market Report 2019: 2018 Results & 2019-2023 Forecasts - Top Competitors Ranking with 30-Year Revenue Analysis." *PR News*, 2 Feb. 2019, www.prnewswire.com/news-releases/united-states-weight-loss--diet-control-market-report-2019-2018-results--2019-2023-forecasts---top-competitors-ranking-with-30-year-revenue-analysis-300803186.html.

11 - Ballard, Jamie . "Exercising More and Eating Healthier Are This Year'S Most Popular New Year's Resolutions." *YouGov*, 12 Dec. 2018, today.yougov.com/topics/society/articles-

reports/2018/12/13/new-years-resolutions-2019-exercise-healthy-eating.

12 - Wolpert , Stuart . "Dieting Does Not Work, UCLA Researchers Report." *UCLA Newsroom*, 3 Apr. 2007, newsroom.ucla.edu/releases/Dieting-Does-Not-Work-UCLA-Researchers-7832.

13 - Hales , Craig, et al. "Prevalence of Obesity and Severe Obesity Among Adults: United States, 2017–2018." *CDC*, www.cdc.gov/nchs/products/databriefs/db360.htm.

14 - CDC. "Normal Weight, Overweight, and Obesity among Adults Aged 20 and over, by Selected Characteristics: United States, Selected Years 1988–1994 through 2013–2016." *CDC*, www.cdc.gov/nchs/data/hus/2017/058.pdf.

15 - Division of Nutrition, Physical Activity, and Obesity. "Defining Adult Overweight & Obesity." *CDC*, 3 June. 2022, www.cdc.gov/obesity/basics/adult-defining.html?CDC_AA_refVal=https%3A%2F%2Fwww.cdc.gov%2Fobesity%2Fadult%2Fdefining.html.

16 - Division of Nutrition, Physical Activity, and Obesity. "About Adult BMI." *CDC*, 3 June. 2022, www.cdc.gov/healthyweight/assessing/bmi/adult_bmi/index.htm

17 - WHO. "The Top 10 Causes of Death." *World Health Organization*, 9 Dec. 2020, www.who.int/news-room/fact-sheets/detail/the-top-10-causes-of-death.

18 - Xu, Hanfei, et al. "Association of Obesity With Mortality Over 24 Years of Weight History: Findings From the Framingham Heart Study." *JAMA Network Open*, vol. 1, no. 7, 2018, pp. e184587–e184587, https://doi.org/10.1001/jamanetworkopen.2018.4587.

19 - Pimenta, Fernanda B. C., et al. "The Relationship Between Obesity and Quality of Life in Brazilian Adults." *Frontiers in Psychology*, vol. 6, 2015, pp. 966–966, https://doi.org/10.3389/fpsyg.2015.00966.

20 - Afshin, Ashkan, et al. "Health Effects of Dietary Risks in 195 Countries, 1990–2017: a Systematic Analysis for the Global Burden of Disease Study 2017." *The Lancet (British Edition)*, vol. 393, no. 10184, 2019, pp. 1958–72, https://doi.org/10.1016/S0140-6736(19)30041-8.

21 - Chen, Phoebe. "Popular, Goal-driven Diets May Lead to Adverse Health Effects, Say UCLA Experts." *Daily Bruin*, 28 Oct. 2019, dailybruin.com/2019/10/28/popular-goal-driven-diets-may-lead-to-adverse-health-effects-say-ucla-experts.

22 - Moss, Michael . "The Extraordinary Science of Addictive Junk Food." *New York Times*, 20 Feb. 2013,

www.nytimes.com/2013/02/24/magazine/the-
extraordinary-science-of-junk-food.html.

23 - Hargrove, James L. "History of the Calorie in Nutrition."
The Journal of Nutrition, vol. 136, no. 12, 2006, pp. 2957–61,
https://doi.org/10.1093/jn/136.12.2957.

24 - Mattes, Richard D., et al. "Impact of Peanuts and Tree
Nuts on Body Weight and Healthy Weight Loss in Adults."
The Journal of Nutrition, vol. 138, no. 9, 2008, pp. 1741–45,
https://doi.org/10.1093/jn/138.9.1741S.

25 - Micha, Renata, et al. "Association Between Dietary
Factors and Mortality From Heart Disease, Stroke, and Type
2 Diabetes in the United States." *JAMA : the Journal of the
American Medical Association*, vol. 317, no. 9, 2017, pp. 912–24,
https://doi.org/10.1001/jama.2017.0947.

26 - Adams, Kelly M., et al. "Status of Nutrition Education in
Medical Schools." *The American Journal of Clinical Nutrition*,
vol. 83, no. 4, 2006, p. 941S–944S,
https://doi.org/10.1093/ajcn/83.4.941S.

27 - Centers for Disease Control and Prevention. "Up to 40
Percent of Annual Deaths from Each of Five Leading US
Causes Are Preventable." *CDC*, 1 May 2014,
www.cdc.gov/media/releases/2014/p0501-preventable-
deaths.html.

28 - National Center for Chronic Disease Prevention and Health Promotion. "Health and Economic Costs of Chronic Diseases." *CDC*, 8 Sept. 2022, www.cdc.gov/chronicdisease/about/costs/index.htm.

29 - Hatori, Megumi, et al. "Time-Restricted Feeding Without Reducing Caloric Intake Prevents Metabolic Diseases in Mice Fed a High-Fat Diet." *Cell Metabolism*, vol. 15, no. 6, 2012, pp. 848–60, https://doi.org/10.1016/j.cmet.2012.04.019.

30 - Lam, Yan Y., and Eric Ravussin. "Analysis of Energy Metabolism in Humans: A Review of Methodologies." *Molecular Metabolism (Germany)*, vol. 5, no. 11, 2016, pp. 1057–71, https://doi.org/10.1016/j.molmet.2016.09.005.

31 - Sumithran, Priya, et al. "Long-Term Persistence of Hormonal Adaptations to Weight Loss." *The New England Journal of Medicine*, vol. 365, no. 17, 2011, pp. 1597–604, https://doi.org/10.1056/NEJMoa1105816.

32 - Kamada, Ikuko, et al. "The Impact of Breakfast in Metabolic and Digestive Health." *Gastroenterology and Hepatology from Bed to Bench*, vol. 4, no. 2, 2011, pp. 76–85, https://doi.org/10.22037/ghfbb.v4i2.127.

33 - Glick, Danielle, et al. "Autophagy: Cellular and Molecular Mechanisms." *The Journal of Pathology*, vol. 221, no. 1, 2010, pp. 3–12, https://doi.org/10.1002/path.2697.

34 - Pearlman, Michelle, et al. "The Association Between Artificial Sweeteners and Obesity." *Current Gastroenterology Reports,* vol. 19, no. 12, 2017, pp. 64–64, https://doi.org/10.1007/s11894-017-0602-9.

35 - Mattson, Mark P., and Rafael de Cabo. "Effects of Intermittent Fasting on Health, Aging, and Disease. Reply." *The New England Journal of Medicine,* vol. 382, no. 18, 2020, pp. 1773–74, https://doi.org/10.1056/NEJMc2001176.

36 - Ozkul, Ceren, et al. "Islamic Fasting Leads to an Increased Abundance of Akkermansia Muciniphila and Bacteroides Fragilis Group: A Preliminary Study on Intermittent Fasting." *The Turkish Journal of Gastroenterology,* vol. 30, no. 12, 2019, pp. 1030–35, https://doi.org/10.5152/tjg.2019.19185.

37 - Carteri, Randhall B., et al. "Intermittent Fasting Promotes Anxiolytic-Like Effects Unrelated to Synaptic Mitochondrial Function and BDNF Support." *Behavioural Brain Research,* vol. 404, 2021, pp. 113163–113163, https://doi.org/10.1016/j.bbr.2021.113163.

38 - Boschmann, Michael, et al. "Water-Induced Thermogenesis." *The Journal of Clinical Endocrinology and Metabolism,* vol. 88, no. 12, 2003, pp. 6015–19, https://doi.org/10.1210/jc.2003-030780.

39 - Wittbrodt, Matthew T., and Melinda millard-stafford. "Dehydration Impairs Cognitive Performance: A Meta-

Analysis." *Medicine and Science in Sports and Exercise*, vol. 50, no. 11, 2018, pp. 2360–68, https://doi.org/10.1249/MSS.0000000000001682.

40 - Murray, Bob, and Christine Rosenbloom. "Fundamentals of Glycogen Metabolism for Coaches and Athletes." *Nutrition Reviews*, vol. 76, no. 4, 2018, pp. 243–59, https://doi.org/10.1093/nutrit/nuy001.

41 - Pontzer, H., et al. "Daily Energy Expenditure through the Human Life Course." *Science,* vol. 373, 2021, pp. 808–812, http://dx.doi.org/10.1126/science.abe5017.

42 - Gormsen, Lars C., et al. "Ketone Body Infusion With 3-Hydroxybutyrate Reduces Myocardial Glucose Uptake and Increases Blood Flow in Humans: A Positron Emission Tomography Study." *Journal of the American Heart Association*, vol. 6, no. 3, 2017, https://doi.org/10.1161/JAHA.116.005066.

43 - Dąbek, Arkadiusz, et al. "Modulation of Cellular Biochemistry, Epigenetics and Metabolomics by Ketone Bodies. Implications of the Ketogenic Diet in the Physiology of the Organism and Pathological States." *Nutrients,* vol. 12, no. 3, 2020, p. 788, https://doi.org/10.3390/nu12030788

44 - Pinto, Alessandro, et al. "Antioxidant and Anti-Inflammatory Activity of Ketogenic Diet: New Perspectives for Neuroprotection in Alzheimer's Disease." Antioxidants,

vol. 7, no. 5, 2018, p. 63,
https://doi.org/10.3390/antiox7050063.

45 - Lopaschuk, Gary D., et al. "Myocardial Fatty Acid
Metabolism in Health and Disease." *Physiological Reviews,*
vol. 90, no. 1, 2010, pp. 207–58,
https://doi.org/10.1152/physrev.00015.2009.

46 - Keon, C. A., et al. "Substrate Dependence of the
Mitochondrial Energy Status in the Isolated Working Rat
Heart." *Biochemical Society Transactions,* vol. 23, no. 2, 1995, p.
307S–307S, https://doi.org/10.1042/bst023307s.

47 - Goodpaster, Bret H., and Lauren M. Sparks. "Metabolic
Flexibility in Health and Disease." *Cell Metabolism,* vol. 25,
no. 5, 2017, pp. 1027–36,
https://doi.org/10.1016/j.cmet.2017.04.015.

48 - Mercola, Joseph. *Fat for Fuel: A Revolutionary Diet to
Combat Cancer, Boost Brain Power, and Increase Your Energy.*
Hay House Inc., 2017.

49 - Mayo Clinic Staff. "Metabolic Syndrome." *Mayo Clinic,* 6
May 2021, www.mayoclinic.org/diseases-
conditions/metabolic-syndrome/symptoms-causes/syc-
20351916.eases-conditions/metabolic-syndrome/symptoms-
causes/syc-20351916

50 - Bikman, Benjamin. *Why We Get Sick. BenBella Books,* 2020.

51 - Pories, Walter J., and Facs G. Lynis Dohm. "Diabetes: Have We Got It All Wrong?: Hyperinsulinism as the Culprit: Surgery Provides the Evidence." *Diabetes Care*, vol. 35, no. 12, 2012, pp. 2438–42, https://doi.org/10.2337/dc12-0684.

52 - Erion, Karel A., and Barbara E. Corkey. "Hyperinsulinemia: a Cause of Obesity?" *Current Obesity Reports*, vol. 6, no. 2, 2017, pp. 178–86, https://doi.org/10.1007/s13679-017-0261-z.

53 - Weiner, M.F. "Rapid Weight-Gain Due to Over-Insulinization." *Obesity & Bariatric Medicine*, vol. 9, no. 4, 1981, pp. 118-119.

54- USDA. *Make Every Bite Count With the Dietary Guidelines.* 9th ed., Dietary Guidelines, 2019.

55 - LeWine, Howard. "Glycemic Index for 60+ Foods." *Harvard Health Publishing*, 16 Nov. 2021, www.health.harvard.edu/diseases-and-conditions/glycemic-index-and-glycemic-load-for-100-foods.

56 - Atkinson, Fiona S., et al. "International Tables of Glycemic Index and Glycemic Load Values: 2008." *Diabetes Care*, vol. 31, no. 12, 2008, pp. 2281–83, https://doi.org/10.2337/dc08-1239.

57 - Harcombe, Zoë, et al. "Evidence from Prospective Cohort Studies Did Not Support the Introduction of Dietary

Fat Guidelines in 1977 and 1983: a Systematic Review."
British Journal of Sports Medicine, vol. 51, no. 24, 2017, pp.
1737–42, https://doi.org/10.1136/bjsports-2016-096409.

58 - Harcombe, Zoë. "Dietary Fat Guidelines Have No
Evidence Base: Where Next for Public Health Nutritional
Advice?" *British Journal of Sports Medicine,* vol. 51, no. 10,
2017, pp. 769–74, https://doi.org/10.1136/bjsports-2016-
096734.

59 - U.S. Department of Agriculture and U.S. Department of
Health and Human Services. *Dietary Guidelines for Americans,
2020-2025.* 9th ed., USDA. December 2020. Available at
https://www.dietaryguidelines.gov/.

60 - de Souza, Russell J., et al. "Intake of Saturated and Trans
Unsaturated Fatty Acids and Risk of All Cause Mortality,
Cardiovascular Disease, and Type 2 Diabetes: Systematic
Review and Meta-Analysis of Observational Studies." *BMJ
(Online),* vol. 351, 2015, pp. h3978–h3978,
https://doi.org/10.1136/bmj.h3978.

61 - Leritz, Elizabeth C., et al. "Elevated Levels of Serum
Cholesterol Are Associated with Better Performance on
Tasks of Episodic Memory." *Metabolic Brain Disease,* vol. 31,
no. 2, 2016, pp. 465–73, https://doi.org/10.1007/s11011-016-
9797-y.

62 - Chung, Chih-Ping, et al. "Associations Between Low
Circulatory Low-Density Lipoprotein Cholesterol Level and

Brain Health in Non-Stroke Non-Demented Subjects."
NeuroImage, vol. 181, 2018, pp. 627–34,
https://doi.org/10.1016/j.neuroimage.2018.07.049.

63 - Teicholz, Nina. *The Big Fat Surprise : Why Butter, Meat,
and Cheese Belong in a Healthy Diet / Nina Teicholz*. First Simon
& Schuster hardcover edition., Simon & Schuster, 2014.

64 - "How Statin Drugs Protect the Heart." *John Hopkins
Medicine*, www.hopkinsmedicine.org/health/wellness-and-
prevention/how-statin-drugs-protect-the-heart.

65 - Laufs, Ulrich, et al. "Clinical Review on Triglycerides."
European Heart Journal, vol. 41, no. 1, 2020, pp. 99–109c,
https://doi.org/10.1093/eurheartj/ehz785.

66-Maihofer, Adam X., et al. "Associations Between Serum
Levels of Cholesterol and Survival to Age 90 in
Postmenopausal Women." *Journal of the American Geriatrics
Society (JAGS)*, vol. 68, no. 2, 2020, pp. 288–96,
https://doi.org/10.1111/jgs.16306.

67 - Gylling, Helena, et al. "Insulin Sensitivity Regulates
Cholesterol Metabolism to a Greater Extent Than Obesity:
Lessons from the METSIM Study." *Journal of Lipid Research*,
vol. 51, no. 8, 2010, pp. 2422–27,
https://doi.org/10.1194/jlr.P006619.

68 - Krok-Schoen, J. L., et al. "Low Dietary Protein Intakes
and Associated Dietary Patterns and Functional Limitations

in an Aging Population: A NHANES Analysis." *The Journal of Nutrition, Health & Aging*, vol. 23, no. 4, 2019, pp. 338–47, https://doi.org/10.1007/s12603-019-1174-1.

69 - Cuenca-Sánchez, Marta, et al. "Controversies Surrounding High-Protein Diet Intake: Satiating Effect and Kidney and Bone Health." *Advances in Nutrition (Bethesda, Md.)*, vol. 6, no. 3, 2015, pp. 260–66, https://doi.org/10.3945/an.114.007716.

70 - Wolfe, Robert R., et al. "Factors Contributing to the Selection of Dietary Protein Food Sources." *Clinical Nutrition*, vol. 37, no. 1, 2018, pp. 130–38, https://doi.org/10.1016/j.clnu.2017.11.017.

71 - Halton, T., and Hu., F.B., "Effects of High Protein Diets on Thermogenesis, Satiety and Weight Loss: A Critical Review." *Journal of the American College of Nutrition*, vol. 23, no. 5, 2004, pp. 373–85, https://doi.org/10.1080/07315724.2004.10719381.

72 - Naghshi, Sina, et al. "Dietary Intake of Total, Animal, and Plant Proteins and Risk of All Cause, Cardiovascular, and Cancer Mortality: Systematic Review and Dose-Response Meta-Analysis of Prospective Cohort Studies." *BMJ*, vol. 370, 2020, pp. m2412–m2412, https://doi.org/10.1136/bmj.m2412.

73 - Saxton, Robert A., and David M. Sabatini. "mTOR Signaling in Growth, Metabolism, and Disease." *Cell*, vol.

168, no. 6, 2017, pp. 960–76,
https://doi.org/10.1016/j.cell.2017.02.004.

74 - Presented by Beach, Rex. "United States Senate
Document #264 Full Version - "MODERN MIRACLE MEN".,
projects.sare.org/wp-content/uploads/united-states-senate-
document-264.pdf.

75 - Hyman, Mark. "Do You Need Supplements?" *Dr.
Hyman*, drhyman.com/blog/2015/04/02/do-you-need-
supplements/.

76 - Ward, Elizabeth. "Addressing Nutritional Gaps with
Multivitamin and Mineral Supplements." *Nutrition Journal*,
vol. 13, no. 1, 2014, pp. 72–72, https://doi.org/10.1186/1475-
2891-13-72.

77 - Vidmar Golja, Maša, et al. "Folate Insufficiency Due to
MTHFR Deficiency Is Bypassed by 5-
Methyltetrahydrofolate." *Journal of Clinical Medicine*, vol. 9,
no. 9, 2020, p. 2836–, https://doi.org/10.3390/jcm9092836.

78 - Vincenti, Alessandra, et al. "Perspective: Practical
Approach to Preventing Subclinical B12 Deficiency in
Elderly Population." *Nutrients*, vol. 13, no. 6, 2021, p. 1913–,
https://doi.org/10.3390/nu13061913.

79 -Mazaheri Nia, Leila, et al. "Effect of Zinc on Testosterone
Levels and Sexual Function of Postmenopausal Women: A
Randomized Controlled Trial." *Journal of Sex & Marital*

Therapy, vol. 47, no. 8, 2021, pp. 804–13,
https://doi.org/10.1080/0092623X.2021.1957732.

80 - Parva, Naveen R., et al. "Prevalence of Vitamin D
Deficiency and Associated Risk Factors in the US Population
(2011-2012)." *Curēus (Palo Alto, CA)*, vol. 10, no. 6, 2018, pp.
e2741–e2741, https://doi.org/10.7759/cureus.2741.

81 - Kumar, Juhi, et al. "Prevalence and Associations of 25-
Hydroxyvitamin D Deficiency in US Children: NHANES
2001-2004." *Pediatrics (Evanston)*, vol. 124, no. 3, 2009, pp.
e362–e370, https://doi.org/10.1542/peds.2009-0051.

82 - Menon, Vikas, et al. "Vitamin D and Depression: A
Critical Appraisal of the Evidence and Future Directions."
Indian Journal of Psychological Medicine, vol. 42, no. 1, 2020,
pp. 11–21, https://doi.org/10.4103/IJPSYM.IJPSYM_160_19.

83 - Pletz, Mathias W., et al. "Vitamin D Deficiency in
Community-Acquired Pneumonia: Low Levels of 1,25(OH)2
D Are Associated with Disease Severity." *Respiratory
Research*, vol. 15, no. 1, 2014, pp. 53–53,
https://doi.org/10.1186/1465-9921-15-53.

84 - Teshome, Amare, et al. "The Impact of Vitamin D Level
on COVID-19 Infection: Systematic Review and Meta-
Analysis." *Frontiers in Public Health*, vol. 9, 2021, pp. 624559–
624559, https://doi.org/10.3389/fpubh.2021.624559.

85 - Carlberg, Carlsten, "Vitamin D: A Micronutrient Regulating Genes." *Current Pharmaceutical Design*, vol. 25, no. 15, 2019; pp. 1740–1746., https://doi.org/10.2174/1381612825666190705193227

86 - Khosravi, Zahra, et al. "Effect of Vitamin D Supplementation on Weight Loss, Glycemic Indices, and Lipid Profile in Obese and Overweight Women: A Clinical Trial Study." *International Journal of Preventive Medicine*, vol. 9, no. 1, 2018, pp. 63–63, https://doi.org/10.4103/ijpvm.IJPVM_329_15.

87 - Brilla, L.R. "Effects of a Novel Zinc-Magnesium Formulation on Hormones and Strength." *Journal of Exercise Physiology*, ISSN An International Electronic Journal vol. 3, no. 4, 2000, pp. 1097–9751.

88 - Baaij, J. H. F. de, et al. "Magnesium in Man: Implications for Health and Disease." *Physiological Reviews*, vol. 95, no. 1, 2015, pp. 1–46, https://doi.org/10.1152/physrev.00012.2014.

89 - Guerrera, Mary P., et al. "Therapeutic Uses of Magnesium." *American Family Physician*, vol. 80, no. 2, 2009, pp. 157–62.

90 - Papanikolaou, Yanni, et al. "U.S. Adults Are Not Meeting Recommended Levels for Fish and Omega-3 Fatty Acid Intake: Results of an Analysis Using Observational Data from NHANES 2003–2008." *Nutrition Journal*, vol. 13,

no. 1, 2014, pp. 31–31, https://doi.org/10.1186/1475-2891-13-31.

91 - Bélanger, Stacey Ageranioti, et al. "Omega-3 Fatty Acid Treatment of Children with Attention-Deficit Hyperactivity Disorder: A Randomized, Double-Blind, Placebo-Controlled Study." *Paediatrics & Child Health,* vol. 14, no. 2, 2009, pp. 89–98, https://doi.org/10.1093/pch/14.2.89.

92 - Su, Kuan-Pin, et al. "Omega-3 Fatty Acids in Major Depressive Disorder: A Preliminary Double-Blind, Placebo-Controlled Trial." *European Neuropsychopharmacology,* vol. 13, no. 4, 2003, pp. 267–71, https://doi.org/10.1016/S0924-977X(03)00032-4.

93 - Gammone, Maria Alessandra, et al. "Omega-3 Polyunsaturated Fatty Acids: Benefits and Endpoints in Sport." *Nutrients,* vol. 11, no. 1, 2018, p. 46–, https://doi.org/10.3390/nu11010046.

94 - Mohajeri, M. Hasan, et al. "Inadequate Supply of Vitamins and DHA in the Elderly: Implications for Brain Aging and Alzheimer-Type Dementia." *Nutrition,* vol. 31, no. 2, 2015, pp. 261–75, https://doi.org/10.1016/j.nut.2014.06.016.

95 - Brenna, J. Thomas. "Efficiency of Conversion of α-Linolenic Acid to Long Chain n-3 Fatty Acids in Man." *Current Opinion in Clinical Nutrition and Metabolic Care,* vol. 5,

no. 2, 2002, pp. 127–32, https://doi.org/10.1097/00075197-200203000-00002.

96 - Plourde, Mélanie, and Stephen C. Cunnane. "Extremely Limited Synthesis of Long Chain Polyunsaturates in Adults: Implications for Their Dietary Essentiality and Use as Supplements." *Applied Physiology, Nutrition, and Metabolism,* vol. 32, no. 4, 2007, pp. 619–34, https://doi.org/10.1139/H07-034.

97 - Jessen, Nadia Aalling, et al. "The Glymphatic System: A Beginner's Guide." *Neurochemical Research,* vol. 40, no. 12, 2015, pp. 2583–99, https://doi.org/10.1007/s11064-015-1581-6.

98 - Medic, Goran, et al. "Short- and Long-Term Health Consequences of Sleep Disruption." *Nature and Science of Sleep,* vol. 9, 2017, pp. 151–61, https://doi.org/10.2147/NSS.S134864.

99 - Ward, Elizabeth M., et al. "Carcinogenicity of Night Shift Work." *The Lancet Oncology,* vol. 20, no. 8, 2019, pp. 1058–59, https://doi.org/10.1016/S1470-2045(19)30455-3.

100 - Longo, Valter D., and Satchidananda Panda. "Fasting, Circadian Rhythms, and Time-Restricted Feeding in Healthy Lifespan." *Cell Metabolism,* vol. 23, no. 6, 2016, pp. 1048–59, https://doi.org/10.1016/j.cmet.2016.06.001.

101 - Daghlas, Iyas, et al. "Sleep Duration and Myocardial Infarction." *Journal of the American College of Cardiology*, vol. 74, no. 10, 2019, pp. 1304–14, https://doi.org/10.1016/j.jacc.2019.07.022.

102 - Chaput, Jean-Philippe, and Angelo Tremblay. "Adequate Sleep to Improve the Treatment of Obesity." *Canadian Medical Association Journal*, vol. 184, no. 18, 2012, pp. 1975–76, https://doi.org/10.1503/cmaj.120876.

103 - Cooper, Christopher B., et al. "Sleep Deprivation and Obesity in Adults: a Brief Narrative Review." *BMJ Open Sport & Exercise Medicine*, vol. 4, no. 1, 2018, pp. e000392–e000392, https://doi.org/10.1136/bmjsem-2018-000392.

104 - Kracht, Chelsea L., et al. "Associations of Sleep with Food Cravings, Diet, and Obesity in Adolescence." *Nutrients*, vol. 11, no. 12, 2019, p. 2899, https://doi.org/10.3390/nu11122899.

105 - Yang, Chia-Lun, et al. "Increased Hunger, Food Cravings, Food Reward, and Portion Size Selection after Sleep Curtailment in Women Without Obesity." *Nutrients*, vol. 11, no. 3, 2019, p. 663–, https://doi.org/10.3390/nu11030663.

106 - Buxton, Orfeu M., et al. "Sleep Restriction for 1 Week Reduces Insulin Sensitivity in Healthy Men." *Diabetes*, vol. 59, no. 9, 2010, pp. 2126–33, https://doi.org/10.2337/db09-0699.

107 - Hirotsu, Camila, et al. "Interactions Between Sleep, Stress, and Metabolism: From Physiological to Pathological Conditions." *Sleep Science*, vol. 8, no. 3, 2015, pp. 143–52, https://doi.org/10.1016/j.slsci.2015.09.002.

108 - Dautovich, Natalie D., et al. "A Systematic Review of the Amount and Timing of Light in Association with Objective and Subjective Sleep Outcomes in Community-Dwelling Adults." *Sleep Health*, vol. 5, no. 1, 2019, pp. 31–48, https://doi.org/10.1016/j.sleh.2018.09.006.

109 - Zheng, Guozhong, et al. "The Effects of High-Temperature Weather on Human Sleep Quality and Appetite." *International Journal of Environmental Research and Public Health*, vol. 16, no. 2, 2019, p. 270, https://doi.org/10.3390/ijerph16020270.

110 - Drake, Christopher, et al. "Caffeine Effects on Sleep Taken 0, 3, or 6 Hours before Going to Bed." *Journal of Clinical Sleep Medicine*, vol. 9, no. 11, 2013, pp. 1195–200, https://doi.org/10.5664/jcsm.3170.

111 - Stutz, Jan, et al. "Effects of Evening Exercise on Sleep in Healthy Participants: A Systematic Review and Meta-Analysis." *Sports Medicine*, vol. 49, no. 2, 2019, pp. 269–87, https://doi.org/10.1007/s40279-018-1015-0.

112 - Oschman, James L., et al. "The Effects of Grounding (earthing) on Inflammation, the Immune Response, Wound Healing, and Prevention and Treatment of Chronic

Inflammatory and Autoimmune Diseases." *Journal of Inflammation Research,* vol. 8, 2015, pp. 83–96, https://doi.org/10.2147/JIR.S69656.

113 - Zschucke, Elisabeth, et al. "The Stress-Buffering Effect of Acute Exercise: Evidence for HPA Axis Negative Feedback." *Psychoneuroendocrinology,* vol. 51, 2014, pp. 414–25, https://doi.org/10.1016/j.psyneuen.2014.10.019.

114 - Dedovic, Katarina, et al. "The Montreal Imaging Stress Task : Using Functional Imaging to Investigate the Effects of Perceiving and Processing Psychosocial Stress in the Human Brain." *Journal of Psychiatry & Neuroscience,* vol. 30, no. 5, 2005, pp. 319–25.

115 - Biddle, Stuart. "Physical Activity and Mental Health: Evidence Is Growing." *World Psychiatry,* vol. 15, no. 2, 2016, pp. 176–77, https://doi.org/10.1002/wps.20331.

116 - Ruegsegger, Gregory N., and Frank W. Booth. "Health Benefits of Exercise." *Cold Spring Harbor Perspectives in Medicine,* vol. 8, no. 7, 2018, p. a029694, https://doi.org/10.1101/cshperspect.a029694.

117 - Stanton, A.M., et al. "The Effects of Exercise on Sexual Function in Women." *Sex Medicine Reviews,* vol. 8, no. 4, 2018, pp. 548–557, https://doi.org/10.1016/j.sxmr.2018.02.004.

118 - Gerbild, Helle, et al. "Physical Activity to Improve Erectile Function: A Systematic Review of Intervention Studies." *Sexual Medicine*, vol. 6, no. 2, 2018, pp. 75–89, https://doi.org/10.1016/j.esxm.2018.02.001.

119 - Westcott, Wayne L. "Resistance Training Is Medicine: Effects of Strength Training on Health." *Current Sports Medicine Reports*, vol. 11, no. 4, 2012, pp. 209–16, https://doi.org/10.1249/JSR.0b013e31825dabb8.

120 - Zhao, Wenjing, et al. "Health Benefits of Daily Walking on Mortality Among Younger-Elderly Men With or Without Major Critical Diseases in the New Integrated Suburban Seniority Investigation Project: A Prospective Cohort Study." *Journal of Epidemiology*, vol. 25, no. 10, 2015, pp. 609–16, https://doi.org/10.2188/jea.JE20140190.

121 - Erickson, Kirk I., et al. "Physical Activity and Brain Plasticity in Late Adulthood." *Dialogues in Clinical Neuroscience*, vol. 15, no. 1, 2013, pp. 99–108, https://doi.org/10.31887/DCNS.2013.15.1/kerickson.

122 - Hart, Peter D., and Diona J. Buck. "The Effect of Resistance Training on Health-Related Quality of Life in Older Adults: Systematic Review and Meta-Analysis." *Health Promotion Perspectives*, vol. 9, no. 1, 2019, pp. 1–12, https://doi.org/10.15171/hpp.2019.01.

123 - Keller, Abiola, et al. "Does the Perception That Stress Affects Health Matter? The Association With Health and

Mortality." *Health Psychology*, vol. 31, no. 5, 2012, pp. 677–84, https://doi.org/10.1037/a0026743.

124 - Lawrence, Elizabeth M., et al. "Happiness and Longevity in the United States." *Social Science & Medicine (1982)*, vol. 145, 2015, pp. 115–19, https://doi.org/10.1016/j.socscimed.2015.09.020.

125 - Rosengren, A., et al. "Stressful Life Events, Social Support, and Mortality in Men Born in 1933." *BMJ*, International edition, vol. 307, no. 6912, 1993, pp. 1102–05, https://doi.org/10.1136/bmj.307.6912.1102.

126 - Yaribeygi, Habib, et al. "The Impact of Stress on Body Function: A Review." *EXCLI Journal*, vol. 16, 2017, pp. 1057–72, https://doi.org/10.17179/excli2017-480.

127 - Yusefzadeh, Hasan, et al. "The Effect of Study Preparation on Test Anxiety and Performance: a Quasi-Experimental Study." *Advances in Medical Education and Practice*, vol. 10, 2019, pp. 245–51, https://doi.org/10.2147/AMEP.S192053.

128 - Uvnäs-Moberg, Kerstin, et al. "Self-Soothing Behaviors with Particular Reference to Oxytocin Release Induced by Non-Noxious Sensory Stimulation." *Frontiers in Psychology*, vol. 5, 2014, pp. 1529–1529, https://doi.org/10.3389/fpsyg.2014.01529.

129 - Sender, Ron, et al. "Revised Estimates for the Number of Human and Bacteria Cells in the Body." *PLoS Biology*, vol. 14, no. 8, 2016, pp. e1002533–e1002533, https://doi.org/10.1371/journal.pbio.1002533.

130 - Hills, Jr, et al. "Gut Microbiome: Profound Implications for Diet and Disease." *Nutrients*, vol. 11, no. 7, 2019, p. 1613–, https://doi.org/10.3390/nu11071613.

131 - Rothschild, Daphna, et al. "Environment Dominates over Host Genetics in Shaping Human Gut Microbiota." *Nature* (London), vol. 555, no. 7695, 2018, pp. 210–28, https://doi.org/10.1038/nature25973.

132 - Turnbaugh, Peter J., et al. "Core Gut Microbiome in Obese and Lean Twins." *Nature*, vol. 457, no. 7228, 2009, pp. 480–84, https://doi.org/10.1038/nature07540.

133 - Ridaura, Vanessa K. Vanessa K., et al. "Cultured Gut Microbiota from Twins Discordant for Obesity Modulate Adiposity and Metabolic Phenotypes in Mice." *Science*, vol. 341, no. 6150, 2013, p. 6150, https://doi.org/10.1126/science.1241214.

134 - Lv, Yanrong, et al. "The Association Between Gut Microbiota Composition and BMI in Chinese Male College Students, as Analysed by Next-Generation Sequencing." *British Journal of Nutrition*, vol. 122, no. 9, 2019, pp. 986–95, https://doi.org/10.1017/S0007114519001909.

135 - "New York University : Americans Are Eating More Ultra-Processed Foods; 18-Year Study Measures Increase in Industrially Manufactured Foods That May Be Contributing to Obesity and Other Diseases." *ENP Newswire*, 2021.

136 - Wang, Lu, et al. "Trends in Consumption of Ultraprocessed Foods Among US Youths Aged 2-19 Years, 1999-2018." *JAMA : the Journal of the American Medical Association*, vol. 326, no. 6, 2021, pp. 519–30, https://doi.org/10.1001/jama.2021.10238.

137 - Zinöcker, Marit, and Inge Lindseth. "The Western Diet–Microbiome-Host Interaction and Its Role in Metabolic Disease." *Nutrients*, vol. 10, no. 3, 2018, p. 365–, https://doi.org/10.3390/nu10030365.

138 - Alcock, Joe, et al. "Is Eating Behavior Manipulated by the Gastrointestinal Microbiota? Evolutionary Pressures and Potential Mechanisms." *BioEssays*, vol. 36, no. 10, 2014, pp. 940–49, https://doi.org/10.1002/bies.201400071.

139 - Bian, Xiaoming, et al. "Gut Microbiome Response to Sucralose and Its Potential Role in Inducing Liver Inflammation in Mice." *Frontiers in Physiology*, vol. 8, 2017, pp. 487–487, https://doi.org/10.3389/fphys.2017.00487.

140 - Abuqwider, Jumana Nabil, et al. "Akkermansia Muciniphila, a New Generation of Beneficial Microbiota in Modulating Obesity: A Systematic Review." *Microorganisms*,

vol. 9, no. 5, 2021, p. 1098–,
https://doi.org/10.3390/microorganisms9051098.

141 - Yaghoubfar, Rezvan, et al. "Modulation of Serotonin
Signaling/metabolism by Akkermansia Muciniphila and Its
Extracellular Vesicles through the Gut-Brain Axis in Mice."
Scientific Reports, vol. 10, no. 1, 2020, pp. 22119–22119,
https://doi.org/10.1038/s41598-020-79171-8.

142 - Shil, Aparna, and Havovi Chichger. "Artificial
Sweeteners Negatively Regulate Pathogenic Characteristics
of Two Model Gut Bacteria, E. Coli and E. Faecalis."
International Journal of Molecular Sciences, vol. 22, no. 10, 2021,
p. 5228, https://doi.org/10.3390/ijms22105228.

143 - Chassaing, Benoit, et al. "Dietary Emulsifiers Impact
the Mouse Gut Microbiota Promoting Colitis and Metabolic
Syndrome." *Nature*, vol. 519, no. 7541, 2015, pp. 92–96,
https://doi.org/10.1038/nature14232.

144 - Ruiz-Ojeda, Francisco Javier, et al. "Effects of
Sweeteners on the Gut Microbiota: A Review of
Experimental Studies and Clinical Trials." *Advances in
Nutrition*, vol. 10, no. 1, 2019, pp. S31–S48,
https://doi.org/10.1093/advances/nmy037.

145 - Cornick, Steve, et al. "Roles and Regulation of the
Mucus Barrier in the Gut." *Tissue Barriers*, vol. 3, no. 1-2,
2015, pp. e982426–e982426,
https://doi.org/10.4161/21688370.2014.982426.

146 - Huang, Ting-Ting, et al. "Current Understanding of Gut Microbiota in Mood Disorders: An Update of Human Studies." *Frontiers in Genetics*, vol. 10, 2019, pp. 98–98, https://doi.org/10.3389/fgene.2019.00098.

147 - LeBlanc, Jean Guy, et al. "Bacteria as Vitamin Suppliers to Their Host: a Gut Microbiota Perspective." *Current Opinion in Biotechnology*, vol. 24, no. 2, 2012, pp. 160–68, https://doi.org/10.1016/j.copbio.2012.08.005.

148 - Laiño, Jonathan Emiliano, et al. "Production of Natural Folates by Lactic Acid Bacteria Starter Cultures Isolated from Artisanal Argentinean Yogurts." *Canadian Journal of Microbiology*, vol. 58, no. 5, 2012, pp. 581–88, https://doi.org/10.1139/w2012-026.

149 - Homayouni Rad, Aziz, et al. "Folate Bio-Fortification of Yoghurt and Fermented Milk: a Review." *Dairy Science & Technology*, vol. 96, no. 4, 2016, pp. 427–41, https://doi.org/10.1007/s13594-016-0286-1.

150 - Mahara, Fenny Amilia, et al. "Folate in Milk Fermented by Lactic Acid Bacteria from Different Food Sources." *Preventive Nutrition and Food Science*, vol. 26, no. 2, 2021, pp. 230–40, https://doi.org/10.3746/pnf.2021.26.2.230.

151 - Rowland, Ian, et al. "Gut Microbiota Functions: Metabolism of Nutrients and Other Food Components." *European Journal of Nutrition*, vol. 57, no. 1, 2018, pp. 1–24, https://doi.org/10.1007/s00394-017-1445-8.

152 - Pandey, Kanti Bhooshan, and Syed Ibrahim Rizvi. "Plant Polyphenols as Dietary Antioxidants in Human Health and Disease." Oxidative Medicine and Cellular Longevity, vol. 2, no. 5, 2009, pp. 270–78, https://doi.org/10.4161/oxim.2.5.9498.

153 - Montagna, Maria Teresa, et al. "Chocolate, 'Food of the Gods': History, Science, and Human Health." *International Journal of Environmental Research and Public Health*, vol. 16, no. 24, 2019, p. 4960, https://doi.org/10.3390/ijerph16244960.

154 - Magrone, Thea, et al. "Cocoa and Dark Chocolate Polyphenols: From Biology to Clinical Applications." *Frontiers in Immunology*, vol. 8, 2017, pp. 677–677, https://doi.org/10.3389/fimmu.2017.00677.

155 - Andújar, Isabel, et al. "Inhibition of Ulcerative Colitis in Mice after Oral Administration of a Polyphenol-Enriched Cocoa Extract Is Mediated by the Inhibition of STAT1 and STAT3 Phosphorylation in Colon Cells." *Journal of Agricultural and Food Chemistry*, vol. 59, no. 12, 2011, pp. 6474–83, https://doi.org/10.1021/jf2008925.

156 - Ahn, Tae-Gue, et al. "Molecular Mechanisms Underlying the Anti-Obesity Potential of Prunetin, an O-Methylated Isoflavone." *Biochemical Pharmacology*, vol. 85, no. 10, 2013, pp. 1525–33, https://doi.org/10.1016/j.bcp.2013.02.020.

157 - Matsui, Naoko, et al. "Ingested Cocoa Can Prevent High-Fat Diet-Induced Obesity by Regulating the Expression of Genes for Fatty Acid Metabolism." *Nutrition*, vol. 21, no. 5, 2005, pp. 594–601, https://doi.org/10.1016/j.nut.2004.10.008.

158 - Melini, Francesca, et al. "Health-Promoting Components in Fermented Foods: An Up-to-Date Systematic Review." *Nutrients*, vol. 11, no. 5, 2019, p. 1189, https://doi.org/10.3390/nu11051189.

159 - Marco, Maria L., et al. "Health Benefits of Fermented Foods: Microbiota and Beyond." *Current Opinion in Biotechnology*, vol. 44, 2016, pp. 94–102, https://doi.org/10.1016/j.copbio.2016.11.010.

160 - Dimidi, Eirini, et al. "Fermented Foods: Definitions and Characteristics, Impact on the Gut Microbiota and Effects on Gastrointestinal Health and Disease." *Nutrients*, vol. 11, no. 8, 2019, p. 1806–, https://doi.org/10.3390/nu11081806.

161 - Tamang, Jyoti Prakash, et al. "Fermented Foods in a Global Age: East Meets West." *Comprehensive Reviews in Food Science and Food Safety*, vol. 19, no. 1, 2020, pp. 184–217, https://doi.org/10.1111/1541-4337.12520.

162 - Chang, Chen-Tien, et al. "Effect of Fermentation Time on the Antioxidant Activities of Tempeh Prepared from Fermented Soybean Using Rhizopus Oligosporus." *International Journal of Food Science & Technology*, Received 7

August 2008; Accepted in revised form 15 December 2008, vol. 44, no. 4, 2009, pp. 799–806, https://doi.org/10.1111/j.1365-2621.2009.01907.x.

163 - Fisberg, Mauro, and Rachel Machado. "History of Yogurt and Current Patterns of Consumption." *Nutrition Reviews*, vol. 73, no. suppl_1, 2015, pp. 4–7, https://doi.org/10.1093/nutrit/nuv020.

164 - Wells, Patricia. "Sauerkraut: It All Began in China." *New York Times*, 14 Nov. 1979, www.nytimes.com/1979/11/14/archives/sauerkraut-it-all-began-in-china.html.

165 - Tamang, Jyoti P., et al. "Editorial: Microbiology of Ethnic Fermented Foods and Alcoholic Beverages of the World." *Frontiers in Microbiology*, vol. 8, 2017, pp. 1377–1377, https://doi.org/10.3389/fmicb.2017.01377.

166 - Rezac, Shannon, et al. "Fermented Foods as a Dietary Source of Live Organisms." *Frontiers in Microbiology*, vol. 9, 2018, pp. 1785–1785, https://doi.org/10.3389/fmicb.2018.01785.

167 - Stiemsma, Leah T., et al. "Does Consumption of Fermented Foods Modify the Human Gut Microbiota?" *The Journal of Nutrition*, vol. 150, no. 7, 2020, pp. 1680–92, https://doi.org/10.1093/jn/nxaa077.

168 - Khalesi S, Bellissimo N, Vandelanotte C, Williams S, Stanley D, Irwin C. A review of probiotic supplementation in healthy adults: helpful or hype? *Eur J Clin Nutr.* 2019 Jan;73(1):24-37. doi: 10.1038/s41430-018-0135-9. Epub 2018 Mar 26. PMID: 29581563.

169 - Khalesi, Saman, et al. "A Review of Probiotic Supplementation in Healthy Adults: Helpful or Hype?" *European Journal of Clinical Nutrition*, vol. 73, no. 1, 2019, pp. 24–37, https://doi.org/10.1038/s41430-018-0135-9.

170 - FAO. "What is Happening to Agrobiodiversity?" *Food and Agriculture Organization of the United Nations*, 1999, www.fao.org/3/y5609e/y5609e02.htm

171 - FAO, "What is Agrobiodiversity?" *Food and Agriculture Organization of the United Nations*, 2004, http://www.fao.org/3/a-y5609e.pdf

172 - Heiman, Mark L., and Frank L. Greenway. "A Healthy Gastrointestinal Microbiome Is Dependent on Dietary Diversity." *Molecular Metabolism*, vol. 5, no. 5, 2016, pp. 317–20, https://doi.org/10.1016/j.molmet.2016.02.005.

173 - Yuan, Xianling, et al. "Gut Microbiota: An Underestimated and Unintended Recipient for Pesticide-Induced Toxicity." *Chemosphere*, vol. 227, 2019, pp. 425–34, https://doi.org/10.1016/j.chemosphere.2019.04.088.

174 - Martin, Michael J., et al. "Antibiotics Overuse in Animal Agriculture: A Call to Action for Health Care Providers." *American Journal of Public Health (1971)*, vol. 105, no. 12, 2015, pp. 2409–10, https://doi.org/10.2105/AJPH.2015.302870.

175 - Smith, Robert P., et al. "Gut Microbiome Diversity Is Associated with Sleep Physiology in Humans." *PloS One*, vol. 14, no. 10, 2019, pp. e0222394–e0222394, https://doi.org/10.1371/journal.pone.0222394.

176 - Appleton, Jeremy. "The Gut-Brain Axis: Influence of Microbiota on Mood and Mental Health." *Integrative Medicine*, vol. 17, no. 4, 2018, pp. 28–32.

177 - Limbana, Therese, et al. "Gut Microbiome and Depression: How Microbes Affect the Way We Think." *Curēus*, vol. 12, no. 8, 2020, pp. e9966–e9966, https://doi.org/10.7759/cureus.9966.

178 - Kelly, John R., et al. "Mood and Microbes: Gut to Brain Communication in Depression." *Gastroenterology Clinics of North America*, vol. 48, no. 3, 2019, pp. 389–405, https://doi.org/10.1016/j.gtc.2019.04.006.

179 - Winter, Gal, et al. "Gut Microbiome and Depression: What We Know and What We Need to Know." *Reviews in the Neurosciences*, vol. 29, no. 6, 2018, pp. 629–43, https://doi.org/10.1515/revneuro-2017-0072.

180 - Xiong, Jiaqi, et al. "Impact of COVID-19 Pandemic on Mental Health in the General Population: A Systematic Review." *Journal of Affective Disorders*, vol. 277, 2020, pp. 55–64, https://doi.org/10.1016/j.jad.2020.08.001.

181 - Banskota, Suhrid, et al. "Serotonin in the Gut: Blessing or a Curse." *Biochimie*, vol. 161, 2019, pp. 56–64, https://doi.org/10.1016/j.biochi.2018.06.008.

182 - Monda, Vincenzo, et al. "Exercise Modifies the Gut Microbiota with Positive Health Effects." *Oxidative Medicine and Cellular Longevity*, vol. 2017, 2017, pp. 3831972–78, https://doi.org/10.1155/2017/3831972.

183 - Fiore, David C., et al. "Antibiotic Overprescribing: Still a Major Concern." The Journal of Family Practice, vol. 66, no. 12, 2017, pp. 730–36.

184 - AAFP. "Antibiotics for Sinusitis." *AAFP*, 1 Jan. 2022, www.fao.org/3/y5609e/y5609e02.htm.

185 - Elvers, Karen T., et al. "Antibiotic-Induced Changes in the Human Gut Microbiota for the Most Commonly Prescribed Antibiotics in Primary Care in the UK: a Systematic Review." *BMJ Open*, vol. 10, no. 9, 2020, pp. e035677–e035677, https://doi.org/10.1136/bmjopen-2019-035677.

186 - Dudek-Wicher, Ruth K., et al. "The Influence of Antibiotics and Dietary Components on Gut Microbiota."

Przegląd Gastroenterologiczny, vol. 13, no. 2, 2018, pp. 85–92, https://doi.org/10.5114/pg.2018.76005.

187 - Park, Jung Ha, et al. "Sedentary Lifestyle: Overview of Updated Evidence of Potential Health Risks." *Korean Journal of Family Medicine*, vol. 41, no. 6, 2020, pp. 365–73, https://doi.org/10.4082/kjfm.20.0165.

188 - Stamatakis, Emmanuel, et al. "Sitting Time, Physical Activity, and Risk of Mortality in Adults." *Journal of the American College of Cardiology*, vol. 73, no. 16, 2019, pp. 2062–72, https://doi.org/10.1016/j.jacc.2019.02.031.

189 - Bressa, Carlo, et al. "Differences in Gut Microbiota Profile Between Women with Active Lifestyle and Sedentary Women." *PloS One*, vol. 12, no. 2, 2017, pp. e0171352–e0171352, https://doi.org/10.1371/journal.pone.0171352.

190 - .Li, Yuanyuan, et al. "The Role of Microbiome in Insomnia, Circadian Disturbance and Depression." *Frontiers in Psychiatry*, vol. 9, 2018, pp. 669–669, https://doi.org/10.3389/fpsyt.2018.00669.

191 - Matenchuk, Brittany A., et al. "Sleep, Circadian Rhythm, and Gut Microbiota." *Sleep Medicine Reviews*, vol. 53, 2020, pp. 101340–101340, https://doi.org/10.1016/j.smrv.2020.101340.

192 - Moloney, Rachel D., et al. "Stress and the Microbiota–Gut–Brain Axis in Visceral Pain: Relevance to Irritable Bowel

Syndrome." *CNS Neuroscience & Therapeutics*, vol. 22, no. 2, 2016, pp. 102–17, https://doi.org/10.1111/cns.12490.

193 - Dangoor, Itzhak, et al. "Specific Changes in the Mammalian Gut Microbiome as a Biomarker for Oxytocin-Induced Behavioral Changes." *Microorganisms*, vol. 9, no. 9, 2021, p. 1938, https://doi.org/10.3390/microorganisms9091938.

194 - Singh, Ajit. "Covid-19: Disinfectants and Sanitisers Are Changing Microbiomes." *BMJ (Online)*, vol. 370, 2020, pp. m2795–m2795, https://doi.org/10.1136/bmj.m2795.

195 - Imhann, Floris, et al. "Proton Pump Inhibitors Affect the Gut Microbiome." *Gut*, vol. 65, no. 5, 2016, pp. 740–48, https://doi.org/10.1136/gutjnl-2015-310376.

196 - Jung, S. B., et al. "Association Between Vitamin B12 Deficiency and Long-Term Use of Acid-Lowering Agents: a Systematic Review and Meta-Analysis." *Internal Medicine Journal*, vol. 45, no. 4, 2015, pp. 409–16, https://doi.org/10.1111/imj.12697.

197 - Vich Vila, Arnau, et al. "Impact of Commonly Used Drugs on the Composition and Metabolic Function of the Gut Microbiota." *Nature Communications*, vol. 11, no. 1, 2020, pp. 362–11, https://doi.org/10.1038/s41467-019-14177-z.

198 - Jackson, Matthew A., et al. "Gut Microbiota Associations with Common Diseases and Prescription

Medications in a Population-Based Cohort." *Nature Communications*, vol. 9, no. 1, 2018, pp. 2655–58, https://doi.org/10.1038/s41467-018-05184-7.

199 -Capurso, Gabriele, and Edith Lahner. "The Interaction Between Smoking, Alcohol and the Gut Microbiome." *Baillière's Best Practice & Research. Clinical Gastroenterology*, vol. 31, no. 5, 2017, pp. 579–88, https://doi.org/10.1016/j.bpg.2017.10.006.

200 - Savin, Ziv, et al. "Smoking and the Intestinal Microbiome." *Archives of Microbiology*, vol. 200, no. 5, 2018, pp. 677–84, https://doi.org/10.1007/s00203-018-1506-2.

201 - Sublette, Marcus G., et al. "Effects of Smoking and Smoking Cessation on the Intestinal Microbiota." *Journal of Clinical Medicine*, vol. 9, no. 9, 2020, p. 2963, https://doi.org/10.3390/jcm9092963.

202 - Shi, Zumin. "Gut Microbiota: An Important Link Between Western Diet and Chronic Diseases." *Nutrients*, vol. 11, no. 10, 2019, p. 2287, https://doi.org/10.3390/nu11102287.

203 - Hills, Jr, et al. "Gut Microbiome: Profound Implications for Diet and Disease." *Nutrients*, vol. 11, no. 7, 2019, p. 1613, https://doi.org/10.3390/nu11071613.

204 - Martínez Steele, Eurídice, et al. "Ultra-Processed Foods and Added Sugars in the US Diet: Evidence from a

Nationally Representative Cross-Sectional Study." *BMJ Open*, vol. 6, no. 3, 2016, pp. e009892–e009892, https://doi.org/10.1136/bmjopen-2015-009892.

205 - Oyagbemi, Ademola Adetokunbo, et al. "Potential Health Benefits of Zinc Supplementation for the Management of COVID-19 Pandemic." *Journal of Food Biochemistry*, vol. 45, no. 2, 2021, p. e13604–n/a, https://doi.org/10.1111/jfbc.13604.

206 - Singh, Akhand Pratap, et al. "Health Benefits of Resveratrol: Evidence from Clinical Studies." *Medicinal Research Reviews*, vol. 39, no. 5, 2019, pp. 1851–91, https://doi.org/10.1002/med.21565.

207 - Matsui, Naoko, et al. "Ingested Cocoa Can Prevent High-Fat Diet-Induced Obesity by Regulating the Expression of Genes for Fatty Acid Metabolism." *Nutrition* , vol. 21, no. 5, 2005, pp. 594–601, https://doi.org/10.1016/j.nut.2004.10.008.

208 - Lambring, Christopher , et al. "Impact of the Microbiome on the Immune System." *Critical Reviews in Immunology*, vol. 39, no. 5, 2020, pp. 313–328, https://doi.org/10.1615%2FCritRevImmunol.2019033233.

209 - Meltzer, David O., et al. "Association of Vitamin D Status and Other Clinical Characteristics With COVID-19 Test Results." *JAMA Network Open*, vol. 3, no. 9, 2020, pp.

e2019722–e2019722,
https://doi.org/10.1001/jamanetworkopen.2020.19722.

210 - WHO. "Cardiovascular Diseases." *World Health Organization*, 1 May 2014,
www.cdc.gov/media/releases/2014/p0501-preventable-deaths.html.

Additional References (used and/or uncited):

1 - Jennifer Petrelli; Kathleen Y. Wolin (2009). *Obesity (Biographies of Disease)*. Westport, Conn: Greenwood. p. 11. ISBN 978-0-313-35275-1.

2 - Chisholm, Hugh, ed. (1911). "Corpulence" . *Encyclopædia Britannica*. 7 (11th ed.). Cambridge University Press. pp. 192–193

3 - Groves, PhD, Barry (2002). "WILLIAM BANTING: The Father of the Low-Carbohydrate Diet". Second Opinions. Retrieved 26 December 2007.

4 - Kawash, Samira (2013). *Candy: A Century of Panic and Pleasure*. New York: Faber & Faber, Incorporated. pp. 185–189. ISBN 9780865477568

5 - Matarese, LE; Pories, WJ (December 2014). "Adult weight loss diets: metabolic effects and outcomes". *Nutrition in Clinical Practice* (Review). 29 (6): 759–67. doi:10.1177/0884533614550251. PMID 25293593.

6 - Flegal KM, Kruszon-Moran D, Carroll MD, Fryar CD, Ogden CL. Trends in obesity among adults in the United States, 2005 to 2014. The Journal of the American Medical Association. 2016;315(21):2284–2291. Available at http://jama.jamanetwork.com/article.aspx?articleid=2526639 External link or

https://www.ncbi.nlm.nih.gov/pubmed/27272580 NIH external link.

7 - Hall KD, et al. Ultra-processed diets cause excess calorie intake and weight gain: A one-month inpatient randomized controlled trial of ad libitum food intake. Cell Metabolism May 16, 2019.

8 - Mortality in the United States, 2018, NCHS Data Brief No. 355, January 2020, https://www.cdc.gov/nchs/products/databriefs/db355.htm

9 - "Obesity and overweight Fact sheet N°311". *WHO*. January 2015.

10 - Strohacker K, Carpenter KC, McFarlin BK. Consequences of Weight Cycling: An Increase in Disease Risk? Int J Exerc Sci. 2009;2(3):191-201. PMID: 25429313; PMCID: PMC4241770.

11 - Kawash, Samira (2013). *Candy: A Century of Panic and Pleasure*. New York: Faber & Faber, Incorporated. pp. 185–189. ISBN 9780865477568.

12 - Painter, Jim ``How Do Food Manufacturers Calculate the Calorie Count of Packaged Foods?". *Scientific American*. July 31, 2006.

13 - D.A.T. Southgate, A.R.C. Food Research Institute, Norwich, UK (October 1981). "The Relationship Between Food composition and Available Energy". *Provisional Agenda Item 4.1.3, Joint FAO/WHO/UNU Expert Consultation on Energy and Protein Requirements, Rome, 5 to 17 October 1981.* Food and Agriculture Organization of the United Nations, World Health Organization, The United Nations University. ESN: FAO/WHO/UNU EPR/81/41 August 1981. Retrieved 9 December 2020.

14 - Cohen P, Barzilai N, Barzilai D, Karnieli E. Correlation between insulin clearance and insulin responsiveness: studies in normal, obese, hyperthyroid, and Cushing's syndrome patients. Metabolism. 1986 Aug;35(8):744-9. doi: 10.1016/0026-0495(86)90242-8. PMID: 3526086.

15 - Woods SC, Decke E, Vasselli JR. Metabolic hormones and regulation of body weight. Psychol Rev. 1974 Jan;81(1):26-43. doi: 10.1037/h0035927. PMID: 4812879.

16 - Cellular respiration. Wikipedia. Retrieved Jan. 11, 2021 https://en.wikipedia.org/wiki/Cellular_respiration

17 - Samarrie, Nadia, Diabetes Health 2013: retrieved January 29, 2021, Scientists Clarify Benefits and Use of Glycemic Index, Load, and Response. https://www.diabeteshealth.com/scientists-clarify-benefits-and-use-of-glycemic-index-load-and-response/

18 - Afaghi A, Ziaee A, Afaghi M. Effect of low-glycemic load diet on changes in cardiovascular risk factors in poorly controlled diabetic patients. *Indian J Endocrinol Metab.* 2012;16(6):991-995. doi:10.4103/2230-8210.103010

19 - From Mendel to epigenetics: History of genetics. Jean Gayon. CR Biol. Jul-Aug 2016;339(7-8):225-30. doi: 10.1016/j.crvi.2016.05.009. Epub 2016 Jun 2.

20 - Nessa Carey, editor. The Epigenetics Revolution: How Modern Biology is Rewriting Our Understanding of Genetics, Disease and Inheritance. 2012. London: Icon Books Ltd.

21 - Teicholz, Nina "The Big Fat Surprise: Why Butter, Meat and Cheese Belong in a Healthy Diet," Simon and Schuster, New York, 2014.

22 - Vij VA, Joshi AS. Effect of 'water induced thermogenesis' on body weight, body mass index and body composition of overweight subjects. J Clin Diagn Res. 2013 Sep;7(9):1894-6. doi: 10.7860/JCDR/2013/5862.3344. Epub 2013 Sep 10. PMID: 24179891; PMCID: PMC3809630.

23 - Leidy HJ, Bossingham MJ, Mattes RD, Campbell WW. Increased dietary protein consumed at breakfast leads to an initial and sustained feeling of fullness during energy restriction compared to other meal times. Br J Nutr. 2009 Mar;101(6):798-803. doi: 10.1017/s0007114508051532. PMID: 19283886.

24 - Leidy HJ, Tang M, Armstrong CL, Martin CB, Campbell WW. The effects of consuming frequent, higher protein meals on appetite and satiety during weight loss in overweight/obese men. Obesity (Silver Spring). 2011 Apr;19(4):818-24. doi: 10.1038/oby.2010.203. Epub 2010 Sep 16. PMID: 20847729; PMCID: PMC4564867.

25 - Petersen, Bente K. and Mark A, Febbraio, "Muscle as an Endocrine Organ: Focus on Muscle-Derived Interleukin-6, American Physiological Society, 01 October 2008, https://doi.org/10.1152/physrev.90100.2007

26 - Yeager, Ashley, "How Exercise Reprograms the Brain," The-Scientist, Nov. 1, 2018. https://www.the-scientist.com/features/this-is-your-brain-on-exercise-64934

27 - Whitham, Martin et al., "Extracellular Vesicles Provide a Means for Tissue Crosstalk during Exercise," Cell Metabolism, 27:1, January 9, 2018. https://doi.org/10.1016/j.cmet.2017.12.001

28 - Venkataramani AS, O'Brien R, Tsai AC. Declining Life Expectancy in the United States: The Need for Social Policy as Health Policy. *JAMA*. 2021;325(7):621–622. doi:10.1001/jama.2020.26339

29 - WHO Global Burden of Disease Study 2010, https://www.who.int/pmnch/media/news/2012/who_burdenofdisease/en/

30 - Iliff JJ, Wang M, Liao Y, Plogg BA, Peng W, Gundersen GA, Benveniste H, Vates GE, Deane R, Goldman SA, Nagelhus EA, Nedergaard M. A paravascular pathway facilitates CSF flow through the brain parenchyma and the clearance of interstitial solutes, including amyloid β. Sci Transl Med. 2012 Aug 15;4(147):147ra111. doi: 10.1126/scitranslmed.3003748. PMID: 22896675; PMCID: PMC3551275

31 - Downie LE, Keller PR, Busija L, Lawrenson JG, Hull CC. Blue-light filtering spectacle lenses for visual performance, sleep, and macular health in adults. *Cochrane Database Syst Rev.* 2019;2019(1):CD013244. Published 2019 Jan 16. doi:10.1002/14651858.CD013244

32 - National Park Service, Timpanogos Cave National Monument, Utah.
https://www.nps.gov/tica/planyourvisit/basicinfo.htm

33 - Breakfast Cereals, from Statistica. Retrieved October 6 2021, https://www.statista.com/outlook/cmo/food/bread-cereal-products/breakfast-cereals/worldwide

34 - Padmanabhan, Geeta, "The Wonder of Water," The Hindu, JANUARY 23, 2011 17:12 IST,
https://www.thehindu.com/features/metroplus/The-wonder-called-water/article15530688.ece\

35 - Ouyang K, Nayak S, Lee Y, et al. Behavioral effects of Splenda, Equal and sucrose: Clues from planarians on

sweeteners. *Neurosci Lett.* 2017;636:213-217.
doi:10.1016/j.neulet.2016.11.017

36 - Mattson MP. Energy intake, meal frequency, and health:
a neurobiological perspective. Annu Rev Nutr. 2005;25:237-
60. doi: 10.1146/annurev.nutr.25.050304.092526. PMID:
16011467.\

37 - Cox CE. Role of Physical Activity for Weight Loss and
Weight Maintenance. *Diabetes Spectr.* 2017;30(3):157-160.
doi:10.2337/ds17-0013

38 - Colberg SR, Sigal RJ, Fernhall B, et al. . Exercise and type
2 diabetes: the American College of Sports Medicine and the
American Diabetes Association joint position statement.
Diabetes Care 2010;33:e147–e167

39 - Amen, Daniel MD, "The World's Best Brain Sport,"
retrieved from website
https://www.danielplan.com/healthyhabits/worldsbestbra
insport/ 8 October 2021.

40 - Schnohr P, O'Keefe JH, Holtermann A, Lavie CJ, Lange
P, Jensen GB, Marott JL. Various Leisure-Time Physical
Activities Associated With Widely Divergent Life
Expectancies: The Copenhagen City Heart Study. Mayo Clin
Proc. 2018 Dec;93(12):1775-1785. doi:
10.1016/j.mayocp.2018.06.025. Epub 2018 Sep 4. PMID:
30193744.

41 - Pericleous P, Stephanides S. Can resistance training improve the symptoms of polycystic ovary syndrome?. *BMJ Open Sport Exerc Med*. 2018;4(1):e000372. Published 2018 Aug 21. doi:10.1136/bmjsem-2018-000372

42 - Di Stefano, Sal The Resistance Training Revolution: The No-Cardio Way to Burn Fat and Age-Proof Your Body in Only 60 Minutes a Week by Sal Di Stefano: April 2021

43 - Levy BR, Slade MD, Kunkel SR, Kasl SV. Longevity increased by positive self-perceptions of aging. J Pers Soc Psychol. 2002 Aug;83(2):261-70. doi: 10.1037//0022-3514.83.2.261. PMID: 12150226.

44 - Ingraham, Christopher, America's top fears: Public speaking, heights, and bugs. The Washington Post, October 30, 2014 https://www.washingtonpost.com/news/wonk/wp/2014/10/30/clowns-are-twice-as-scary-to-democrats-as-they-are-to-republicans/

45 - Takac M, Collett J, Blom KJ, Conduit R, Rehm I, De Foe A. Public speaking anxiety decreases within repeated virtual reality training sessions. *PLoS One*. 2019;14(5):e0216288. Published 2019 May 31. doi:10.1371/journal.pone.0216288

46 - Jessica Bayes, Nitish Agrawal, and Janet Schloss. The Journal of Alternative and Complementary Medicine. Feb 2019.169-180. http://doi.org/10.1089/acm.2018.0086

47 - Fairfield KM, Fletcher RH. Vitamins for chronic disease prevention in adults: scientific review. JAMA. 2002 Jun 19;287(23):3116-26. doi: 10.1001/jama.287.23.3116. Erratum in: JAMA 2002 Oct 9;288(14):1720. PMID: 12069675.

48 - Nair R, Maseeh A. Vitamin D: The "sunshine" vitamin. *J Pharmacol Pharmacother*. 2012;3(2):118-126. doi:10.4103/0976-500X.95506

49 - Yamanaka R, Tabata S, Shindo Y, et al. Mitochondrial Mg(2+) homeostasis decides cellular energy metabolism and vulnerability to stress. *Sci Rep*. 2016;6:30027. Published 2016 Jul 26. doi:10.1038/srep30027

50 - Lim LS, Mitchell P, Seddon JM, Holz FG, Wong TY. Age-related macular degeneration. *Lancet*. 2012 May 5;379(9827):1728-38. doi: 10.1016/S0140-6736(12)60282-7. PMID: 22559899.

51 - Zhu B, Wang X, Li L. Human gut microbiome: the second genome of human body. *Protein Cell*. 2010 Aug;1(8):718-25. doi: 10.1007/s13238-010-0093-z. Epub 2010 Aug 28. PMID: 21203913; PMCID: PMC4875195.

52 - Sharma A, Amarnath S, Thulasimani M, Ramaswamy S. Artificial sweeteners as a sugar substitute: Are they really safe?. *Indian J Pharmacol*. 2016;48(3):237-240. doi:10.4103/0253-7613.182888

53 - Rowland I, Gibson G, Heinken A, et al. Gut microbiota functions: metabolism of nutrients and other food components. *Eur J Nutr*. 2018;57(1):1-24. doi:10.1007/s00394-017-1445-8

54 - Rooks MG, Garrett WS. Gut microbiota, metabolites and host immunity. *Nat Rev Immunol*. 2016;16(6):341-352. doi:10.1038/nri.2016.42

55 - Marco ML, Heeney D, Binda S, Cifelli CJ, Cotter PD, Foligné B, Gänzle M, Kort R, Pasin G, Pihlanto A, Smid EJ, Hutkins R. Health benefits of fermented foods: microbiota and beyond. Curr Opin Biotechnol. 2017 Apr;44:94-102. doi: 10.1016/j.copbio.2016.11.010. Epub 2016 Dec 18. PMID: 27998788.

56 - Dimidi E, Cox SR, Rossi M, Whelan K. Fermented Foods: Definitions and Characteristics, Impact on the Gut Microbiota and Effects on Gastrointestinal Health and Disease. *Nutrients*. 2019;11(8):1806. Published 2019 Aug 5. doi:10.3390/nu11081806

57 - Melini F, Melini V, Luziatelli F, Ficca AG, Ruzzi M. Health-Promoting Components in Fermented Foods: An Up-to-Date Systematic Review. *Nutrients*. 2019 May 27;11(5):1189. doi: 10.3390/nu11051189. PMID: 31137859; PMCID: PMC6567126.

58 - Alcock J, Maley CC, Aktipis CA. Is eating behavior manipulated by the gastrointestinal microbiota?

Evolutionary pressures and potential mechanisms. *Bioessays*. 2014;36(10):940-949. doi:10.1002/bies.201400071

59 - Ahmad SY, Friel J, Mackay D. The Effects of Non-Nutritive Artificial Sweeteners, Aspartame and Sucralose, on the Gut Microbiome in Healthy Adults: Secondary Outcomes of a Randomized Double-Blinded Crossover Clinical Trial. Nutrients. 2020 Nov 6;12(11):3408. doi: 10.3390/nu12113408. PMID: 33171964; PMCID: PMC7694690.

60 - Ahola, A.J., Lassenius, M.I., Forsblom, C. *et al*. Dietary patterns reflecting healthy food choices are associated with lower serum LPS activity. *Sci Rep 7*, 6511 (2017). https://doi.org/10.1038/s41598-017-06885-7

61 - Ramanan D, Cadwell K. Intrinsic Defense Mechanisms of the Intestinal Epithelium. *Cell Host Microbe*. 2016;19(4):434-441. doi:10.1016/j.chom.2016.03.003

62 - Salehi B, Mishra AP, Nigam M, et al. Resveratrol: A Double-Edged Sword in Health Benefits. *Biomedicines*. 2018;6(3):91. Published 2018 Sep 9. doi:10.3390/biomedicines6030091

63 - Worrall G. Acute sinusitis. *Can Fam Physician*. 2011;57(5):565-567.

64 - Katzmarzyk PT, Powell KE, Jakicic JM, Troiano RP, Piercy K, Tennant B, et al. Sedentary Behavior and Health:

update from the 2018 Physical Activity Guidelines Advisory Committee. *Med Sci Sports Exerc.* 2019;51:1227–41.

65 - Maihofer AX, Shadyab AH, Wild RA, LaCroix AZ. Associations between Serum Levels of Cholesterol and Survival to Age 90 in Postmenopausal Women. J Am Geriatr Soc. 2020 Feb;68(2):288-296. doi: 10.1111/jgs.16306. Epub 2020 Jan 13. PMID: 31930739.

Made in the USA
Las Vegas, NV
20 September 2024

95482778R00223